SHOULD I BE TESTED
FOR CANCER?

SHOULD I BE TESTED FOR CANCER?

Maybe Not and Here's Why

H. GILBERT WELCH, M.D., M.P.H.

UNIVERSITY OF CALIFORNIA PRESS
Berkeley   Los Angeles   London

University of California Press
Berkeley and Los Angeles, California

University of California Press, Ltd.
London, England

© 2004 by the Regents of the University of California

Library of Congress Cataloging-in-Publication Data

Welch, H. Gilbert.
    Should I be tested for cancer? : maybe not and here's why /
H. Gilbert Welch.
        p.   cm.
    Includes bibliographical references and index.
    ISBN 0-520-23976-8 (cloth : alk. paper)
        1. Cancer—Popular works.   2. Cancer—Diagnosis—Popular
works.   3. Medical screening—Popular works.   I. Title.
    RC263 .W43   2003
    616.99'4075—dc21   2003012771

Manufactured in the United States of America
12   11   10   09   08   07   06   05   04
10   9   8   7   6   5   4   3   2   1

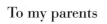

To my parents

CONTENTS

ACKNOWLEDGMENTS

There are few truly original ideas in either science or medicine. Instead, most of us contribute to scholarship in small steps—perhaps by taking a slightly different tack within an established field or by transferring an idea from one field (or application) to another.

The idea that trying to find early cancer might not always help people did not originate with me. I was first introduced to the notion early in my career at Dartmouth when a faculty mentor suggested that I work with a new member of the radiology faculty, Bill Black. Bill exposed me to the two general problems caused by early diagnosis of any disease: (1) more people are told they are sick, and (2) the average patient *appears* to do better—even if treatment is useless or harmful. We went on to document these problems for physicians in a special article in the *New England Journal of Medicine.* Although Bill would be the first to point out that neither of these ideas originated with him (he would put Alan Morrison at the top of the list and would also credit Alvan Feinstein, Tony Miller, and John Bailar, among others), it is not an overstatement to say that Bill is the colleague who has had the most profound effect on my career and ultimately is most responsible for my writing this book.

As anyone who has tried it knows, however, writing a book takes a lot more than an idea. A critical ingredient is time. I am indebted to my hospital, the Department of Veterans Affairs Medical Center in White River Junction, Vermont—and in turn, to our director and chief of staff—for providing me with that time. The key was then to get out of town—away from my day-to-day faculty duties—and to acquire an office with desk, an internet connection, and a phone that didn't ring. In the 2001–2002 academic year I was able to achieve these conditions in Lyon, France, while a visiting scientist at the International Agency for Research on Cancer, the cancer section of the World Health Organization. It was during this year that the bulk of this book was written. I am grateful for the hospitality extended to me and my family by colleagues there and for the kindness of many other Lyonnais. I am also very appreciative for three sources of salary support that made the year possible: the Department of Veterans Affairs, the Helmut Schumann Special Fellowship in Healthful Living, and the Visiting Scientist Award from the International Agency for Research on Cancer.

Getting ideas down on paper is one thing; the discipline of revision so that others can easily understand them is another. I am indebted to my parents for appreciating this distinction: to my father who instilled in me the value of writing well and to my mother who made it clear I couldn't do it on the first pass. Although neither participated directly in this work, both influenced me greatly. Special thanks go to Jeanne West for the direct contribution of regularly reading, editing, questioning, and critiquing chapters e-mailed from Lyon. My wife, Linda, also provided valuable feedback, but more important has been her steadfast support of my work over the years. There is much I would not have done without her.

H. Gilbert Welch
Thetford, Vermont

The conventional wisdom
about cancer testing
and what this book is about

Everybody knows someone who has had cancer. My father died of cancer when I was in medical school. His sister died of cancer. So did my mother-in-law. Two of my next-door neighbors have had cancer. One of my closest high school buddies just learned he has cancer. Six friends and family members: my experience is probably not dissimilar from yours. There seems to be a lot of cancer out there, and that is scary.

We are all scared of cancer. It has the reputation of being a horrible disease—a part of your own body gone hopelessly awry. It grows uncontrollably. It spreads in mysterious and unexpected ways. It eats away at normal tissue. It ultimately weakens and kills its host.

Even doctors are scared of cancer. I was reminded of this when attending one of my colleague's lectures on disease prevention at Dartmouth Medical School. John has always been known for giving informative but humorous lectures, and this was no exception. He was showing a series of *New Yorker* cartoons mocking the national obsession with avoiding heart disease. One showed a panting jogger being scrutinized by two bystanders. One remarks to the other, "I hear exercise doesn't really help you live longer, it only seems that way." Another had a group of middle-aged people sitting in a living room littered with giant chunks of cheese with one explaining to a visitor: "We were hoping the cholesterol would kill the mice." A third depicted a nurse running down a hospital corridor, pursued by a number of large heartlike blobs and shouting, "Run! It's a heart attack!" The medical students loved it; they were howling.

"Its interesting how we have learned to joke about the most common cause of death in our society [heart disease]," John continued, "but what if all these cartoons were about cancer?" The room went dead. You could feel the tension. A cartoon with a caption, "Run! It's a breast cancer!"? Not funny. Each student seemed to be struggling with the contradiction. So was I. How could cancer possibly be funny? It was one of the most powerful classroom moments I have ever experienced.

There is something different about cancer. It is no joking matter. It is common and it is scary. We naturally want to do everything we can to avoid getting it. That's why we are all interested in cancer prevention— and why it can be such an emotional topic.

CONVENTIONAL APPROACH TO CANCER PREVENTION

There are two basic strategies for preventing cancer: health promotion and early detection. Health promotion means encouraging such healthy behaviors as regular exercise, sun protection, a balanced diet, and not smoking. Early detection means testing: the use of sophisticated technologies to find early cancers that are then removed. You will note that this strategy is not really about preventing cancer; rather, it is about finding cancer early.

Compared to health promotion, early detection has a lot of appeal. No one has to make a difficult lifestyle change; instead, health care professionals do something to you. They take pictures of the inside of your body. They draw your blood. They remove a piece of your tissue. They use high-tech machines. It is a scientific process, a concrete service, and it leads to an "answer." From the doctors' perspective, early detection has other appealing features: ordering a test is quick and easy, and it has an established billing process—unlike health promotion counseling. Not surprisingly, early detection has become the dominant cancer prevention strategy in mainstream American medicine.

To be fair, our diagnostic technology *is* pretty impressive. Doctors can manipulate flexible fiber-optic devices and look for cancer in our lungs, stomach, or large intestine. We can detect molecules in the blood that suggest the presence of liver or prostate cancer, even when there are very few of these molecules around—"few" as in one billionth of a gram per milliliter of blood (comparable to finding one or two grains of sand in a large bucket of soil). We can detect genetic abnormalities that increase the risk of getting a number of cancers—changes in human DNA itself, the molecular basis of heredity. But most impressive is what we can see when radiation, sound waves, magnetic fields, and particle physics are combined with massive computing power in our scanning machines. Using the images made by CAT scans, ultrasound scans, MRI scans, and PET scans, radiologists are able to detect subtle structural defects deep inside the body. These scans can take pictures of the human body as often as every millimeter of thickness, then have a computer reconstruct images and rotate them in any plane for a 3-D effect. Frankly, both patients and doctors alike are enamored by what our diagnostic technology can see.

So we test for cancer—a lot. Each year millions of Americans undergo mammograms to look for breast cancer, colonoscopies to look for colon cancer, PSA tests to look for prostate cancer, Pap smears to look for cervical cancer, and MRIs and CAT scans to look for a broad range of other cancers. Although traditionally ordered by doctors, these tests can now be ordered by consumers, allowing them to bypass the intermediate step of consulting a health care provider. People can even order a "complete body scan" over the Internet to detect cancers in the brain, lung, and abdomen.

The conventional wisdom is that all this testing is good. The idea is simple: cancer grows and spreads to distant parts of the body. When cancer is this far along it is really hard to treat. But if doctors catch cancer earlier, before it spreads, it is much easier to treat. It's a familiar idea: fix small problems before they become big ones. In other words, the conventional wisdom is that looking for early cancer always makes sense—it can only help. The answer to the question "Should I get tested for cancer?" seems like a no-brainer: of course you should.

In this book, I will articulate a different view. The reality is not so simple. Although the effort to find cancer early can be beneficial, it can also hurt. For there is another side to trying to find cancer early: tests can be wrong, people are made to worry unnecessarily, some are treated unnecessarily, and some are even harmed by treatment.

Let me be clear: I'm not going to tell you never to be tested for cancer. That would be too simple. Instead, I am going to urge caution. I will suggest that you be a little skeptical of claims that testing saves lives. I will recommend that you ask hard questions. And I will encourage you to think about what really matters to you. In short, I will argue that a decision to forgo cancer testing can be a reasonable option.

This flies in the face of medical dogma. And because cancer is such a scary disease, this message may not be very comforting. It does not inspire confidence that doctors know exactly what they are doing. It does not lead to a simple solution. For these reasons, it is not a message that I delight in communicating. But I believe it is an important message, particularly as we develop more and more tests and find more and more abnormalities. And I believe that understanding the two sides of early detection will help people make better choices, and be less likely to be hurt physically and emotionally by the testing and treatment process.

At the very least, I hope to persuade you that there are reasons to think twice when someone proposes more testing. Some will argue that if it makes sense to test for cancer X every five years, it makes even better sense to test every six months. Or that if it makes sense to test 50- to 70-year-olds for cancer Y, it would be even better to test 20- to 90-year-olds. Or that if it makes sense to do genetic tests on people with a strong family history of cancer, it would be even better to do genetic tests on everybody. I will argue that more testing will always create more problems but may not produce additional benefit. I also hope to demonstrate how someone who proposes less testing may be motivated by something other than saving money for insurance companies.

WHO THIS BOOK IS (AND IS NOT) FOR

One of my favorite editorials ever to appear in a medical journal was by a Tennessee physician and was entitled "The Last Well Person."[1] It is a short story that takes place in the not-too-distant future. The lone character is a 53-year-old professor of freshman algebra at a small college in the Midwest. Despite extensive medical evaluation, no doctor has been able to find anything wrong with him. But he is the only remaining person for whom this is true. Although it is just a story, the author warned that "if the behavior of doctors and the public continues unabated, eventually every well person will be labeled as sick." I share his concern.

Looking for cancer has become a cultural norm. Americans are being regularly tested for cancer: 20 million men for prostate cancer, 30 million men and women for colon cancer, 37 million women for breast cancer, and over 90 million women for cervical cancer.[2] And in the future, millions more may contemplate undergoing tests that are still under development, particularly DNA tests looking for cancer genes.

This book is for those individuals who are open to questioning the wisdom of these testing efforts. While the topic may be particularly relevant to health professionals, health care policymakers, and social scientists, it is also relevant to anyone who is still healthy. Because as you will soon see, one way to become sick is to start looking for something to be wrong.

Let me be equally clear about who this book is *not* for. It is not for people who are sick. More precisely, it is not for people who have symptoms of cancer. It is not for women who have a breast mass or abnormal uterine bleeding. It is not for men who have a testicular mass. It is not for individuals of either sex who have a change in bowel habits or have difficulty swallowing or who feel like their stomach gets full after eating just a little food. These people should seek medical care and should be tested for cancer. And it is not meant for people who know they have cancer. This book is not about what to do if you know you have cancer; it is about informing the decision of whether to look for cancer when you are well.[3]

It's also not a book for people who need to have simple answers. None of us likes uncertainty—but this book is full of it. Given the uncertainties, different people will (and should) make different decisions. In fact, the same person could make different decisions about different cancer tests—and different decisions at different times of life. This is because cancer is a complex disease, and medicine a complex field. If you prefer to believe that medicine is a perfectly understood science, practiced by infallible and all-knowing professionals, then this book is not for you.

Finally, this book is not for people who are looking for an excuse to trash mainstream (some say Western) medicine. It is not an exposé about the horrors of modern medical practice, nor is it intended to dissuade people from seeing a doctor when they are sick. Furthermore, it is not intended to persuade people never to be tested or never to be treated for cancer. Medicine *can* help, and real progress has been made in cancer treatment. But there are real problems with early cancer diagnosis, despite the best intentions. Understanding these problems will help guide your relationship with preventive medical care and ensure that it fits your needs.

WHAT IS CANCER?

Cancer can occur in any organ in the body; however, cancer is much more common in some organs than others (although this varies from country to country). Table 1 gives a sense of the most important cancers in the United States. The column labeled "Number of new cases" lists the top five most commonly diagnosed cancers; the "Number of deaths" column lists the cancers responsible for the most deaths in the country. The "Years of life lost" column requires a little explanation, for it combines two factors: (1) how many people died and (2) at what age they died. A cancer death in a 40-year-old woman, for example, represents about 42 years of life lost (because the typical 40-year-old woman is expected to live to age 82). A cancer death in an 80-year-old woman, on the other hand, represents about nine years of life lost (because the typical 80-year-old woman is expected to live to age 89).[4] So if two cancers cause roughly the same number of deaths, but one generally causes death in younger people, it is ranked higher in this column.

The relative positions of cancers in Table 1 actually tell quite a lot about the various cancers. Skin cancer is the most common form of cancer, but

Table 1   Top five cancers in terms of numbers of new cases,
deaths, and years of life lost in the United States, 2003

Rank	Number of new cases	Number of deaths	Years of life lost
1	Skin	Lung	Lung
2	Prostate	Colon	Breast
3	Breast	Breast	Colon
4	Lung	Pancreatic	Pancreatic
5	Colon	Prostate	Leukemia

SOURCE: http://SEER.cancer.gov.

most skin cancers are not deadly. That is why skin cancer does not appear in the other two columns. Lung cancer may not be the most common cancer, but more people die of it than of any other cancer (in fact, more than from breast, prostate, and colon cancer combined). Prostate cancer is the second most common form of cancer, but it often doesn't cause death. And because it is generally a disease of older men, prostate cancer is not in the top five in terms of years of life lost. Breast and colon cancer, which are relatively common, frequently cause death, and often occur in the middle of life, appear in all three columns.

But just knowing where and how often cancer occurs does not answer the question "What is cancer?" Although it is a simple question, there is no simple answer. Indeed, the word *cancer* encompasses a broad spectrum of disorders, making the cancer/not cancer distinction fuzzy. Because this complexity is responsible for many of the problems outlined in this book, I want to begin by attempting to define cancer.

Let's start with the dictionary. Mine reads, "Cancer: a malignant tumor of potentially unlimited growth that expands locally by invasion and systematically by metastasis." *Malignant* in turn means "tending to infiltrate, metastasize, and terminate fatally," while *metastasis* (or the verb *metastasize*) refers to the spread of disease to a distant site. My medical dictionary is a little more terse, defining cancer as "a cellular tumor the natural course of which is fatal."

This is the way most of us think about cancer. It is bad. It grows relentlessly (local invasion). It pops up in unexpected places (metastasis). It spreads throughout the body. And it kills you. If cancer is thus defined, it seems logical that it must be found and it must be treated.

But doctors diagnose almost all cancer before people die from it, and they diagnose most cancer before any metastasis occurs. So the diagnosis can be made without the foregoing criteria, that is, without death and without metastasis. There must be another definition for cancer, then, and there is: the microscopic definition.

The diagnosis of cancer is made by pathologists—those physicians who specialize in the performance of laboratory tests and the examination of human tissue under the microscope. Physicians who are worried about a cancer diagnosis generally take a piece of the organ in question (a biopsy) and send it to the lab. The pathologist then examines thin sections of the tissue under the microscope.

The microscopic definition depends on the appearance of individual cells. The less individual cells look like the normal cells found in the organ, the more likely they are cancer. The more individual cells vary in size and shape, the more likely they are cancer. And the more the pathologist sees individual cells in the midst of dividing, the more likely they are cancer.

The microscopic definition also depends on the appearance of the collection of cells—the architecture that results from how individual cells fit together. Growths that are clearly walled off from surrounding tissue, as if in a cocoon, are less likely to be cancer. Conversely, growths that extend into surrounding tissue and invade nearby blood vessels are more likely to be cancer.

So again: what is cancer? Is it the lethal disease that has spread throughout the body, or is it the microscopic abnormality seen in a group of cells?

You might reasonably ask, "What's the difference? People who develop the microscopic abnormality are bound to develop the lethal disease if they are not treated." In fact, sometimes that is true, but sometimes it is not.

The natural course of untreated cancer—what epidemiologists call the "natural history"—turns out to be highly variable. Cancer is a dynamic process that may proceed in many different ways. You might envision the process as involving steps, beginning with a cell that has suffered some genetic damage:

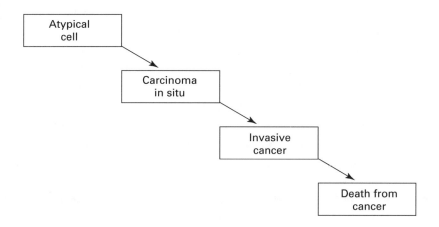

But the process may proceed at very different speeds, and it may even be stopped by the body's immune system. So what pathologists call cancer in fact encompasses a broad range of entities that may evolve in very different ways. Some may grow very fast, others may grow very slowly, and a few may even go away. This heterogeneity in the natural history of cancer is the explanation for many of the problems raised in this book: why tests miss some cancers, why there are others you would rather not know about, why it's hard to know who really has early cancer, and why our cancer statistics can be so misleading.

AN OVERVIEW OF WHAT IS COMING

Each chapter in Part I of this book details a different problem. Chapter 1 explains why testing is unlikely to help you. The basic point is simple: since most people who are tested will never get cancer, most people cannot benefit from testing. And others will die from cancer despite our best efforts to find cancer early. In fact, screening tests tend to miss the fastest-

growing and most deadly cancers. So while some may believe that anyone who didn't get tested and dies of cancer would have been saved had
they had the test, that simply is not true, as the major studies of cancer
testing detailed in this chapter show. And when you see how many people
die from something else altogether, you may conclude that the benefit of
testing is much smaller than you previously realized.

Chapter 2 reviews what is probably the most familiar problem of cancer testing: patients with abnormal screening tests often do not have cancer. But before they are pronounced cancer free, they may have to go
through multiple tests—some of which are invasive, unpleasant, and risk
serious complications. Some may even get trapped in a seemingly endless cycle of testing. And throughout the entire process, people suffer the
emotional toll of wondering whether or not they have cancer. In this chapter I review the data on the frequency of "cancer scares" following mammograms, PSA tests for prostate cancer, Pap smears, and take-home fecal
occult blood tests for colon cancer. You will see how one test often begets
another, thereby increasing the chance of a cancer scare.

Chapter 3 introduces a much less familiar problem: tests cause people
to receive unnecessary treatment. Here I introduce an idea that might be
hard to believe, which is that some cancers don't need treatment. These
cancers may grow so slowly that people die of other causes long before
their cancer causes symptoms, or they may not grow at all. Both situations are examples of pseudodisease: cancers that will never matter to patients. Because doctors can never be sure who has pseudodisease and who
has a true disease, we tend to treat everybody. Patients with pseudodisease cannot benefit from treatment, however, because they were never going to develop symptoms of cancer in the first place. Instead they experience the emotional burden of a cancer diagnosis and face the side effects,
complications, and risk of death associated with cancer therapies. And
the only way patients get diagnosed with pseudodisease is by having a
test looking for early cancer. In this chapter I present the evidence that
pseudodisease exists in a number of cancers, particularly breast and
prostate cancer.

Chapter 4 deals with the other implication of pseudodisease: there are
cancers you would rather not know about. For years autopsies have found

"surprise" cancers in people who died from something else. Now, with the help of our advanced diagnostic technologies, we are finding these cancers during life. In this chapter I examine the data from autopsy studies that suggest there is a reservoir of undetected cancer in people not known to have cancer during life—because the cancer they had never bothered them. The existence of this reservoir means the harder we look, the more we find, and the more likely it is that the cancers found are pseudodisease—the cancers for which treatment is worse than the disease.

Chapter 5 describes a problem that doctors have yet to come to grips with: pathologists don't always agree about who has cancer. This is in part because the diagnosis of cancer is based on subjective judgments about cells as they appear under the microscope. But it is also because the cancer/noncancer distinction is blurrier than any of us would like. The problem is not that pathologists disagree about big, obvious cancers that are invading surrounding tissue, but that they disagree about the subtle abnormalities—the very abnormalities most commonly identified with screening. In this chapter I review the literature on the differing diagnoses of pathologists, which in turn exposes a fundamental problem of early cancer detection: doctors do not have a reliable way to diagnose early cancer.

Chapter 6 postulates a fundamentally different problem with cancer testing, relating to the cost of competing agendas. In the past, doctors saw patients without having a preset agenda. Now increasingly we have one, and much of it is related to cancer screening tests. From the physician's perspective, screening has a lot of appeal: it is a concrete service, and it identifies actionable problems. Discussing patient concerns, in contrast, can feel ethereal and frequently concludes with sympathy rather than an actionable plan. Given the limited time for clinic visits, these two tasks may compete. The more time we spend ordering, communicating, and following up on abnormal test results, the less time we spend dealing with what you want to talk about. In Chapter 6 I speculate about this downside of screening and leave you with the problem as I see it: worrying too much about what may matter in the future distracts your doctor from what matters now.

In Part II, I move on to topics intended to help you be a better-educated consumer of cancer testing. Chapter 7 explores the culture of medicine and the forces that promote cancer testing. This is about more than just money. Doctors have a tendency to appreciate technology and see medicine as continually improving—an attitude that reinforces the use of new tests. Although some see using the newest test as protection against malpractice suits, most doctors want to use new tests because we think patients want them. But other forces promote cancer testing as well. Health care managers do so because it's good public relations, and test developers have a professional interest in demonstrating that new tests are worth doing. Because proponents have such strong interests, I encourage healthy skepticism in assessing the information you are given about tests.

In Chapter 8 I introduce the three basic numbers doctors use to measure cancer and cancer treatments: incidence—how frequently people develop cancer; mortality—how frequently they die from it; and five-year survival rates. Because testing is changing the way we count cancer, though, these statistics can fool us—particularly five-year survival. In this chapter I introduce the numbers and go over examples of them being used incorrectly to illustrate what to look out for in news reports about new screening tests.

In Chapter 9 I try to convey the limits of medical research, using various investigations of mammography as a case study. You will see that, while it is relatively easy to figure out whether a treatment helps sick patients, it is very difficult to learn whether testing helps healthy people. A well-designed study of a cancer screening test takes many years, thousands of participants, and millions of dollars. And even then the answer may not be definitive. Although many look to genetic testing to be a breakthrough against cancer, in truth a genetic test will at best help doctors estimate the probability that an individual will develop a lethal cancer. The test can never be definitive: it can't tell you that you will or will not get cancer. Instead genetic tests only address risk—raising more questions about *when, whether,* and *how* to look for cancer. In this chapter I explain why there will likely always be more questions than answers.

The final chapter deals with the question of how to move forward. There is no right answer about cancer screening, only a strategy that works for you individually. I provide suggestions to help you develop that strategy—suggestions that will help you give your doctor permission not to test and that will help you know what questions to ask your doctor and, more important, what questions to ask yourself.

A FINAL NOTE REGARDING LANGUAGE

Before moving on, I feel obliged to make a few comments on word choice. Although occasionally I use the broader term *health care provider,* for simplicity I use the term *doctor* more frequently. This is not meant to exclude other health care givers. On the contrary, it is important to acknowledge that physician assistants and nurse practitioners are assuming larger and more important roles in medicine—particularly in the delivery of primary care (where much cancer testing is initiated).

Then there is a pair of words having different meanings that I'll nonetheless use interchangeably throughout the book: cancer "screening" and cancer "testing." One is a very precise term, the other pretty broad. Although I can hear the howls of protest from screening experts in my mind, this muddling of words is intentional. Let me explain: *Screening* is the precise term. Formally, it means the systematic examination of asymptomatic people to detect and treat disease. Obviously we cannot screen for every disease (or you would spend your life in a doctor's office). So experts tend to prioritize the settings in which they advocate screening using three criteria. First, the disease has to be relatively common (we do not screen millions of people to find a handful of cases). Second, the disease must be bad (we do not screen for colds). Finally, the disease must be somehow less treatable when symptoms appear than when detected early (we do not screen for pneumonia). One breast cancer screening expert summed up the last criterion by saying, "Screening is always a second best, an admission of failure of prevention or treatment."[5]

Cancer, in general, meets all three of these criteria: it is common, it frequently leads to death, and our treatment of most advanced cancers does not work very well. So we screen for cancer. Remember the two fundamental characteristics of screening: (1) it involves people without symptoms and (2) it is systematic, there is a plan for the population. It is from studying these organized screening efforts that we have learned about some of the unintended side effects of early diagnosis.

In the real world of modern medicine, however, screening is not the only way doctors find early cancers. We also find a fair amount of cancer in the course of testing for something else. There is nothing systematic about this process; we kind of stumble on it. A man comes to the doctor's office with back pain, the doctor orders a CAT scan of his back, and the radiologist finds a cancer in the kidney. The back pain had nothing to do with the cancer but everything to do with *finding* the cancer. Or a woman comes in with chest pain after falling on the ice, the urgent care provider gets a chest X-ray to check for broken ribs, and the radiologist finds lung cancer. The chest pain had nothing to do with the cancer but, again, everything to do with finding the cancer. It is luck, good or otherwise.

For obvious reasons, this is called serendipitous detection. The more we test, for whatever reason, the more serendipitous cancer detection will occur. But strictly speaking, that is not screening. So I'll often use the broader term *cancer testing* so as to include all of the ways we detect cancer early. Because whether or not testing is part of a systematic effort, testing can create problems.

Finally, I want to mention a phrase you will not see a lot in this book: basic principles. It's too dry, too theoretical. Instead I will talk about problems—problems that could happen to you. And I will talk about how the problems relate to testing for specific cancers. You will hear a lot about testing for prostate and breast cancer—two cancers for which debate about screening is most public. You will also learn about cancer testing that has been accepted for decades (cervical cancer), one recommended more recently (colon cancer), and one where the promotion is ongoing (lung cancer). And you will hear about testing for cancers you may rarely hear about (renal cell carcinoma, melanoma, and neuroblastoma). Behind all these specific examples are general problems. And because they stem from basic principles of cancer testing, these problems are bound to occur with any cancer test—even those not yet developed.

PART I

PROBLEMS YOU SHOULD KNOW ABOUT

ONE   *It is unlikely that you will benefit*

Most people have had some experience with cancer screening. Your parents may have been tested for cancer. You may have been tested yourself—particularly if you are female—because almost all women have had at least one Pap smear, the test for cancer of the cervix. And you may know people who have had small cancers detected by screening tests—particularly in the breast and prostate, where the chances are good that small cancers will be found.

On the surface, it all seems simple enough: screening tests find early cancers. People who have early cancers do better than people with advanced cancers. Screening tests can prevent advanced cancers. Screening saves lives.

Unfortunately, it is not that simple. In this chapter, I summarize what we know about the benefits of screening for cancer and review some of the major studies of screening. But what I most want to do is give you some perspective on the size of the benefit you might expect from cancer screening—under the best conditions.

The fact is that even the best screening test will have only a limited effect. One reason is that most people who are tested will never get cancer, and people who will never get cancer do not benefit from cancer screening. But there is another reason for the limited effect of screening, which is that even with an ideal test, some people will die of cancer anyway.

Let's begin with an unfortunate reality: screening tends to miss the worst cancers.

CANCERS MISSED BY SCREENING

Many of my regular patients can be described as old-time Vermonters—rugged, elderly men who have spent most of their lives outdoors (and because I work for the Department of Veterans Affairs, all of my patients have spent some portion of their life in the military). One of my favorite patients still works, at age 77. It's hard work, too: drilling water wells. He has an old drilling rig that uses a winch to wind up a metal cable that, in turn, lifts a tremendous weight maybe 25 feet in the air. The entire rig shimmies a little bit under the load. When the weight is released, it drops and smashes into the well casing below. The process is repeated over and over, slowly banging the casing into the ground. Heavy weights, taut metal cables, extreme forces . . . it's the kind of thing I like to watch from a distance. Suffice it to say, this man's primary health concern has not been cancer.

Nevertheless, we have discussed prostate cancer screening. I told him that while we have studies that show some screening tests work, such as mammography for breast cancer and fecal occult blood for colon cancer, we also know that some, like chest X-rays for lung cancer, do not. I added that many tests have never been rigorously studied, including the blood test for prostate cancer, which measures prostate specific antigen (better known as PSA). He had participated in a study in which patients watched a video developed by some of my colleagues that laid out what physicians do and do not know about the PSA test. For him the decision about whether to have the test was easy: he didn't want it. He even went on to appear in a television documentary on PSA testing, serving as one member of a pair of patients who made opposite decisions about having the test.

But a few years later he came to the clinic and was not his usual joyful self. Typically he would manage to find the bright side of things and would punctuate our conversations with wonderful hearty laughter. I had never seen him teary before and asked him what was wrong. He told me that his daughter in Connecticut had been diagnosed with breast cancer a few months previously. The cancer was now all over her lungs. She had had a mammogram just three months before the diagnosis. He thought I had said that mammography was one of the tests that had been proven to work. Now he wanted to know why the screening test had missed the cancer.

SCREENING AND CANCER DYNAMICS

Screening is the name given to the effort to find disease in people who are well (that is, who have no symptoms of the disease being sought). In cancer, the effort typically involves testing people at regular intervals. The idea behind cancer screening is familiar: if you "catch" cancer before symptoms appear, it will be easier to treat. At least two conditions are assumed by this statement: (1) that tests can find early cancers, and (2) that early treatment works better than late treatment. Let's focus on the finding part first.

In the last two decades our ability to find things has increased exponentially. Today we can detect subtle changes in the body's chemistry that suggest cancer simply by drawing a vial of blood (tests for such antigens as PSA, alpha fetoprotein for liver cancer, and CA 125 for ovarian cancer). Structural abnormalities the size of a pea can be found virtually anywhere in the body using MRI and CAT scans. And mammograms can detect the earliest forms of breast cancer, appearing as tiny collections of calcium that are only slightly larger than this period.

So how could a mammogram miss a breast cancer that a few months later was already widely metastatic—that is, had spread throughout this man's daughter's lungs? Perhaps it was bad technology, a technically poor mammogram. Or perhaps it was a bad radiologist, who missed an obvious cancer. But I bet it was bad cancer, a cancer that was growing very fast. Unfortunately, this is the kind of cancer that screening tests are most likely to miss.

To understand why screening tends to miss the fastest-growing cancers, consider how cancer detection relates to cancer dynamics. Because cancer begins with an abnormal cell and grows over time, there is a window of opportunity during which a screening test can potentially detect it.[1] This time period, theoretically at least, starts with the abnormal cell. It ends when the patient notices that something is wrong—that is, when the cancer causes symptoms. Once a cancer causes symptoms, there is no reason to screen for cancer. People with symptoms go to the doctor with a complaint, and any testing done in this context represents diagnosis, not screening.

This window of opportunity for early cancer detection is known as the preclinical phase and can be illustrated as follows:

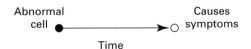

Next consider the fact that cancers grow at different rates. A fast-growing cancer causes symptoms early; a slow-growing cancer causes symptoms only after a considerable period of time. The preclinical phases for a fast and a slow cancer could be represented something like this:

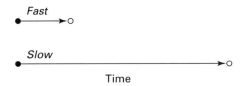

So the faster a cancer is growing, the shorter its preclinical phase. And fast-growing cancers are the most deadly: they are the ones we would most like to catch with cancer testing.

Add to this the fact that we don't screen everybody every day. So even if our tests were perfect, we'd miss some cancers simply because we did not test at the right time. But which ones will be missed?

To answer that, I want to show you a more involved illustration, one that maps the preclinical phase for 12 cancers:

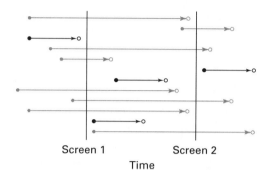

Screen 1   Screen 2
Time

Note that the cancers start at different times and grow at different rates. The vertical lines denote the time of screening tests; when the arrow intersects the line, the cancer is detected early (that is, before the cancer becomes symptomatic). Note that all four missed cancers (dark arrows) had short preclinical phases; in other words, they were fast-growing cancers. Thus, of the six fast-growing cancers (short arrows), only two were detected by the screening test. Sure, this is a constructed hypothetical example, but the basic principle is simple: it's hard for a screening test to catch a fast-growing cancer because the opportunity to do so is so brief. On the other hand, screening tests are good at detecting slow-growing cancers.

So my bet is that my patient's daughter had a very fast growing cancer. Her situation highlights the irony of cancer screening: the cancers we would most like to catch are also the cancers that are most likely to become apparent (that is, produce symptoms) in the interval between screening tests. Cancers that appear in between screening tests are called interval cancers. They are known to be among the most aggressive cancers.

Of course, the missed breast cancer might have been avoided by more frequent screening. We could conceivably test every day, but it will soon become clear why none of us would want that—even without considering the time and money involved.

The reality is that there is a limit to what we can expect any cancer screening test to do. Screening tests will always tend to miss the deadliest cancers. So even if a screening program could catch 90 percent of all cancers, we would still be lucky if it could prevent 50 percent of the cancer deaths, simply because the missed cancers *are* so deadly. And in fact, none of the screening tests that have been studied are even that good.

TESTING THE TESTS

Although it is easy to know whether a test can find early cancers, it is harder to know whether early treatment really helps people. It is tempting to compare people who chose to be screened with people who were not screened, but these groups differ in many important ways other than the simple decision to be tested. In particular, people who choose to be screened tend to be better educated, wealthier, and more attentive to health in general (more likely to exercise, less likely to smoke). So while this kind of comparison is convenient, it is not fair. People who choose to be screened are bound to do better than others simply because they are healthier—even if the screening test doesn't help one bit.

To avoid this problem, researchers need to perform an experiment in which study participants are assigned to one of two groups solely on the basis of chance—essentially by flipping a coin. In this way, the group assigned to screening will be very similar to that assigned to no screening. This allocation process is called randomization; this kind of study is called a randomized trial.

There are three cancers for which screening has been given this kind of scrutiny: lung cancer, breast cancer, and colorectal cancer. Not surprisingly, these are the three cancers responsible for the most years of life lost in the United States. Let me briefly summarize the findings of these randomized trials.

The best-studied screening test, with eight major randomized trials, is mammography, the X-ray technique used to detect breast cancer. Despite this high level of scrutiny, there is still plenty of debate about its benefit (as we'll see in Chapter 9). The typically quoted figure, however, is that middle-aged women who have the test regularly reduce their chance of dying from breast cancer by about a third.[2]

Three randomized trials of fecal occult blood testing for colon cancer have been carried out. This test is performed at home: a person smears a small portion of a bowel movement on a special card provided by his or her doctor. After three are completed, the cards are sent to the lab and tested for trace amounts of blood. The presence of blood on any card may be a sign of colon cancer (but more often is not). The three randomized trials have shown that this screening test can reduce the chance of dying from colon cancer by about 15 to 30 percent.[3]

There have also been three randomized trials of chest X-ray screening for lung cancer. Each focused on the group of people most likely to get the disease: smokers. These randomized trials have shown that regular chest X-rays do not change the chance of dying from lung cancer. Consequently, no one currently recommends chest X-ray screening.[4]

That's where we are right now. We have good studies on only three screening tests. Two work, neither perfectly. Neither even prevents 50 percent of the deaths from the cancer in question.

Why? First, the screening tests tend to miss the most aggressive forms of the disease—the problem of interval cancers discussed earlier. Two mammography trials in Sweden, for example, found that women who developed interval cancers were more than twice as likely to die of breast cancer than were women who had breast cancer detected on a mammogram.[5] Second, some of the people whose cancer is detected by screening die from cancer anyway. In the Swedish trials, over half of the breast cancer deaths were among women whose cancers were found by mammography. Nevertheless, mammography and fecal occult blood testing appear to be able at least to reduce your chance of dying from cancer.

YOUR CHANCE OF DYING FROM CANCER

Note that this discussion about reducing your chance of dying from cancer hasn't yet touched on what your chance of dying from cancer actually *is*. That's pretty typical. In the promotion of screening, health care providers tend to talk about screening using numbers that express relative reductions (e.g., "Your chances of dying are 20 percent less"; "You are one-third less likely to die") and never mention the risk itself—what scientists call the absolute risk.

What is your absolute risk of dying from cancer? The answer depends on the cancer and how old you are. Out of a group of a thousand 60-year-old women, for example, nine will die of breast cancer in the next 10 years. That sentence states an absolute risk. Another way to express the same risk is to say that for an average 60-year-old woman, the chance of dying from breast cancer in the next 10 years is 9 in 1,000.[6] An absolute risk is always calculated as the chance of a specific event occurring within a specific time period. Here, when I speak of absolute risk, I use it to mean the chance of death occurring within the next 10 years.

Where do these numbers come from? The federal government carefully compiles data on virtually all deaths in the United States. This national death index includes information on both the age of death and the cause of death, as well as gender. So for any one age and gender we know how many people died each year and why. To calculate the absolute risk of dying of breast cancer in the next 10 years for a 60-year-old woman thus involves adding the number of breast cancer deaths among 60-year-olds, 61-year-olds, and on up to 69-year-olds, then dividing by the total number of women turning age 60. For the whole country, the approximate numbers are 90,000 breast cancer deaths over 10 years among 10 million women turning age 60, or 9 per 1,000.[7]

Now let's move to consider the benefit of screening. (Note that in the following calculations I have purposely erred on the side of overstating benefit—so think of these numbers as the best case.) If an average 60-year-old woman has a 9-in-1,000 chance of dying from breast cancer in the next 10 years, and screening, under the most optimistic scenario, lowers that chance by a third, her chances of dying from breast cancer if she undergoes regular mammography drop to 6 in 1,000. In other words, the net effect of screening for 60-year-old women is an absolute reduction in the chance of breast cancer death by 3 in 1,000. Because the risk of cancer is lower in 50-year-olds, for this group the benefit of mammography is somewhat smaller.

In other words, the number of deaths avoided changes with age. This is easy to see if the data are presented in a list, answering the question "In the next 10 years, out of 1,000 American women, how many will die of breast cancer? (And how many will avoid death because of screening?)"

Age	Die from breast cancer *without* mammography	Die from breast cancer *with* mammography	Avoid death *because of* mammography
50	6	4	2
60	9	6	3
70	13	8.5	4.5

In the case of fecal occult blood testing, let's focus on men because men have a slightly higher risk for colon cancer at every age than women. Again I address the question "In the next 10 years, out of 1,000 American men, how many will die of colon cancer? (And how many will avoid death because of screening?)"—and again I use the optimistic assumption that screening lowers the chance of dying from colon cancer by a third.

Age	Die from colon cancer *without* fecal occult blood testing	Die from colon cancer *with* fecal occult blood testing	Avoid death *because of* fecal occult blood testing
50	3	2	1
60	8	5	3
70	15	10	5

The numbers aren't that different from those for breast cancer. Colon cancer death in men is a little less common than breast cancer death in women at the younger ages, and it's a little more common at older ages. But the number of deaths avoided is just about the same.

One of the reviewers of this book looked at these charts and thought some important data were missing: although they show how many people benefit from screening, they do not show how many people receive no benefit. She thought I needed another column. Here's what the chart would look like for fecal occult blood testing:

Age	Die from colon cancer *without* fecal occult blood testing	Die from colon cancer *with* fecal occult blood testing	Avoid death *because of* fecal occult blood testing	Receive *no benefit from* fecal occult blood testing
50	3	2	1	999
60	8	5	3	997
70	15	10	5	995

And of course, the new column would look just about the same for mammography. No doubt about it: the vast majority of people do not benefit from either test.

To be perfectly fair, I should be clear that this result is typical for any population-based effort to prevent a particular disease, such as cancer screening. The reason is simple: a person can only benefit if he or she is destined to get the disease in question—and most people are not.

So, when we talk about screening in terms of relative reductions in breast or colon cancer mortality, we obscure some important absolute numbers. In fact, the upper limit of benefit from either fecal occult blood testing or mammography is the prevention of 5 deaths per 1,000 individuals screened over 10 years. You will have to decide whether a benefit of this size—and indeed, calculated using a best-case scenario—is large enough to accept the problems associated with testing (discussed in subsequent chapters).

A TALE OF TWO TRIALS

To give a little more perspective on the benefit of screening, I will share with you some more in-depth information about two randomized trials: the Health Insurance Plan of New York Study (hereafter referred to as the HIP study), which assessed mammography; and the Minnesota Colon

Cancer Control Study (the Minnesota study), which evaluated fecal occult blood testing.[8]

A word on why I selected these two trials. First, they both had among
the most favorable results for screening. Second, they are both "classic
studies," which means doctors refer to them a lot. And finally, while all
the other trials of mammography and fecal occult blood testing took place
in Europe or Canada (where it could be argued that health care is practiced differently), these two studies were done in the United States.[9]

The HIP study was started in the early 1960s by one of the nation's
oldest prepaid health plans. Roughly 60,000 women aged 40 to 64 were
randomly allocated into two equal-sized groups: one that received mammograms and one that continued with usual medical care, which at that
time did not include mammography. After about 10 years of follow-up,
192 women had died of breast cancer in the no-mammography group, versus 147 in the mammography group. In other words, of 30,000 women
who were screened for a 10-year period, 147 died of breast cancer despite
screening, while an estimated 45 (192 minus 147) avoided a breast cancer
death because of screening.

The Minnesota study began in the late 1970s and included both women
and men. Roughly 45,000 participants aged 50 to 80 were randomly allocated to one of three equal-sized groups: one that was tested for fecal blood
every year, one that was tested every other year, and a no-testing group.
For simplicity, I'm going to ignore the middle group here. After about 13
years of follow-up, 121 in the no-testing group had died of colon cancer,
versus 82 in the annual-testing group. Thus of 15,000 men and women
who were screened annually for 13 years, 82 died of colon cancer despite
screening, while an estimated 39 (121 minus 82) avoided a colon cancer
death because of screening.

The reason for all these numbers is to present a realistic perspective on
the magnitude of the benefit from the two screening tests we know the
most about. To illustrate the numbers, Figure 1 presents the death rates[10]
for the target cancer in the two studies, breast and colon cancer, with and
without testing.

Even these numbers are incomplete because they are just about deaths
from cancer. Think for a minute about why you might want to be screened.

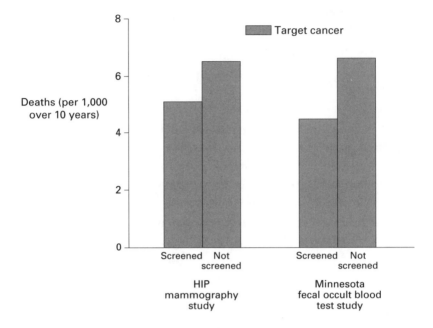

Figure 1.   Death rate for target cancer (*left,* breast cancer; *right,* colon cancer) in the two U.S. randomized trials of screening.

Is it because you want to reduce your chance of a cancer death? Or is it because you want to reduce your chance of death, period?

Some will be quick to point out that we all die. While I have used the shorthand "chance of dying" in the above discussion, I really mean mortality rate: the number of people who die over a specified time period. Many mortality rates can be calculated, including colon cancer mortality, heart disease mortality, and overall mortality—the chance of death in general. To come at it from a different perspective, then, let me ask: If you were considering a new screening test, which question would you be more interested in? (1) Does screening reduce mortality from the target cancer? or (2) Does screening reduce overall mortality?

Let's go back to the HIP and Minnesota studies, both of which kept track of all deaths. In Figure 2, each trial is represented by a pair of columns: one for the group that was screened and one for the group that was not

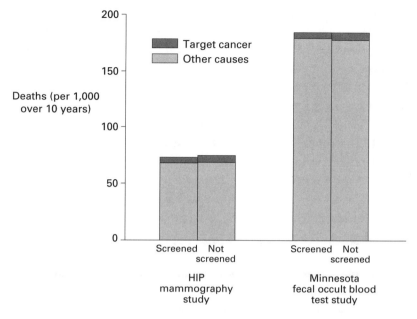

Figure 2.   Death rate for all causes in the two U.S. randomized trials of screening.

screened. The dark stripes on top of the columns represent the mortality rate for the target cancer (the same information shown in the first graph, although the perspective has changed). The larger, lightly shaded area underneath is the mortality rate from causes other than the target cancer. The two together—that is, the entire height of the column—is the rate of death in general: overall mortality.

What do you make of this graph? You may be struck first by the fact that the biggest difference is between the two studies themselves. Participants were much less likely to die in the HIP study than in the Minnesota study. But this doesn't tell you anything about mammography and fecal occult blood testing; it simply reflects the fact that a group of women aged 40 to 64 died at a lower rate than a group of men and women aged 50 to 80. No surprise there. As people grow older, they are more likely to die.

What may surprise you about this graph is that most of the deaths in these studies in fact had nothing to do with the cancers being targeted. Another way to say this is that mortality from the target cancer (breast cancer or colon cancer) is a relatively small portion of overall mortality. Furthermore, mammograms and fecal occult blood testing affect only a small portion of that portion.

The most vexing question is whether overall mortality has really changed. For the HIP study, I think the answer is yes.[11] As such, I think the HIP study probably represents the best-case effect of breast cancer screening: a reduction in breast cancer mortality (that's the difference in the width of the black stripes) and no change in mortality from other causes. As a result, overall mortality was lower for the screened group. Assuming the study was performed well (a topic discussed in Chapter 9), this is good news: the chance of dying has fallen.

For the Minnesota study, I'm not sure what to think. Colon cancer mortality fell in the screened group, but the mortality from other causes actually increased. In particular, people in the screened group had more deaths from heart disease. This could be chance, or it could be a side effect of the screening process. Consider that 15,000 people were being screened, many of whom were aged and frail (in fact, more than 3,000, or 20 percent of the screened group, died in the course of the study). At least 5,000 had an extensive evaluation of their colon, an evaluation that includes emptying the bowel with a cathartic, some anesthesia, and often minor surgery. All it would take is for 39 of these people to have a fatal heart attack as a consequence of any aspect of the procedure, and the benefit of avoiding 39 colon cancer deaths is canceled out. It's a conjecture; no one really knows how to explain the increase in mortality from other causes. But there is no doubt about one thing: overall mortality remained unchanged in the screened group.

Because the HIP study shows only a very small reduction in overall mortality in the screened group, and the Minnesota study shows none at all, you might wonder whether the benefits of screening are being overstated to the general public. Is it really fair to suggest that mammograms are "the chance of a lifetime"? Is it justified to scare healthy people with a sign saying, "The early warning signs of colon cancer: You feel great. You have a healthy appetite. You're only 50" in order to promote colorectal cancer screening? I think not. The data simply do not warrant this kind of enthusiasm.

SUMMARY

Some believe that anyone who dies of cancer and wasn't screened would have been saved had they had a test. But that's not true. Sometimes cancers appear in the interval between screening tests. These interval cancers are growing rapidly and are more deadly than cancers detected by screening. Other times cancers are found by screening but people still die from the disease. Clearly, screening helps only in certain cases.

In order to find those cases, a lot of people have to be screened. The vast majority of people will not have cancer. They can't be helped by the screening test. Even with our best screening tests, therefore, the benefit is limited. Given this limited benefit, readers will understand how downsides might become important to consider.

You might think I am trying to persuade you not to have a mammogram or not to undergo fecal occult blood testing. I'm not. Again, these two tests probably help people. Buried in the statistics are a few people who benefited greatly, people who beat cancer and wouldn't have otherwise.[12] But I object to the emerging mindset that patients should be persuaded, frightened, and coerced into undergoing these tests. There is today a certain "medical correctness" about screening—making patients feel guilty if they choose not to pursue testing. This is wrong.

You might be wondering about all the screening tests we haven't talked about. What about PSA tests for prostate cancer? What about ultrasounds for ovarian cancer? What about Pap smears for cervical cancer? What about skin exams for melanoma? What about head scans for cancers of the brain? What about body scans for cancer in the abdomen? No randomized trials have been carried out for any of these tests. They may help people. They may have little effect (other than expense). Or they may set off a chain of events that ultimately hurts more people than it helps. And there will be even more screening tests to wonder about in the future.

In this chapter, I have illustrated that there is only so much benefit to be had from cancer testing. Because it will always tend to miss the fastest-growing cancers, screening can only reduce mortality from cancer by so much. And because any given cancer is a relatively rare cause of death in general, cancer screening can at best have a small impact on overall mortality. Whenever the benefit is small, the downsides of testing become more important. They are the subject of the next five chapters.

TWO   *You may have a "cancer scare"*
       and face an endless cycle of testing

In our society, information gathering is viewed almost uniformly as a good thing. (It *is* the "information age," after all.) Nowhere is this more true than in medicine. For doctors, more information is always better. In the past, most of our information came from the patient. Now it increasingly comes from machines.

Doctors like tests because we see them as objective and more reliable than our own subjective judgments. We also see tests as something tangible we can offer the patient at the end of a clinic visit. Patients like tests for the same reasons.[1] Ordering a test validates their concerns and promises concrete information—a definitive diagnosis. Sometimes patients even perceive their care as substandard if they are not given some sort of test. While doctors and patients recognize that treatments may have side effects or lead to complications, both tend to view testing as something that can only help. The prevailing attitude seems to be *It can't hurt just to gather a little information.*

Of course, that is not always true. In this chapter I describe the most familiar problem with cancer testing: the test can be wrong. In short, people with abnormal screening tests often don't have cancer. But before they find out for sure, they may have to go through multiple tests—tests that may be unpleasant and that may lead to complications. Throughout the testing period, they will worry about whether they have cancer. And some may never get a definitive answer. That can hurt a lot.

TRAPPED IN AN ENDLESS CYCLE OF TESTING

Every other week I see patients in the Veterans Administration walk-in clinic, a clinic for patients who either don't have an appointment or don't have a doctor. I recently saw a gentleman who wanted to have his cholesterol tested. He also wanted to talk about PSA screening for prostate cancer. Like many of our veterans, he came into the examination room accompanied by his wife. Both were in their early 70s.

His cholesterol was fine. I asked him what he'd like to know about prostate cancer screening, and he said he wanted to know why there was any debate as to its usefulness. Just by knowing there was a debate, he was further along than many. I said we really didn't know whether it saved lives or not. He said, "What's the harm in trying?" I told him that many older men have elevated PSAs (because of enlarged prostate glands) and yet don't have prostate cancer. But the only way they can find out that they don't have cancer is to have a prostate biopsy (a procedure no one enjoys—more on that later). I also mentioned that some people have indeterminate biopsy results: they won't be told they have cancer, but they also won't be told they do not.

His wife, who had been listening quietly, now spoke up: "It's like ASCUS, isn't it?"

I was stunned. I was talking about the ambiguities of PSA screening for prostate cancer; she thought immediately of Pap smear screening for cervical cancer. It was a remarkable connection, one many doctors might miss. And she was right. ASCUS stands for "atypical squamous cells of unknown significance," which are frequently detected in a Pap smear. It's not cancer, but it's not normal. Instead we call it an "indeterminate" result. I told her the analogy was right on target.

She and her husband then shared what she had been through over the past five years. She had been told that her Pap smear was abnormal. It was then repeated every three to six months. She had had a colposcopy: an optical instrument was placed in the vagina to better visualize the cervix. She had been biopsied. She had been told she did not have cancer. But the Pap smears were still abnormal. She had had cryocauterization: a cold probe was used to freeze and kill cells on the cervix. She had had laser therapy: a high energy light beam was used to burn and kill cervical cells. Most recently she had had a cervical conization: a procedure in which the core of the cervix is cut out. Her Pap smear was still abnormal.

Some doctors were suggesting that she have a hysterectomy—removal of her entire uterus and cervix—even though they could not prove she had cancer. Others were saying she should just keep checking. Neither approach appealed to her. She was fed up. What she wanted was the answer to an apparently simple question: "Is there a problem or not?"

TESTS ARE IMPERFECT

In an ideal world, we'd have ideal tests. They'd be cheap, simple, safe, and quick. And they would never be wrong. Among people who had cancer, the test for cancer would always be positive, while among those who didn't have cancer, the test would always be negative. Positive tests could immediately be followed by early treatment; negative tests would result in immediate reassurance. This utopian ideal would look something like this:

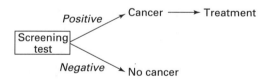

Cancer, however, is a diagnosis made by examining human tissue under the microscope. And the only way to look at tissue under the microscope is to do a biopsy: cut a small piece of tissue and remove it from the body. A biopsy is a small operation, and like any operation, it can be disruptive and painful and can lead to complications. So it's not the kind of test you want to perform on everyone.

The job of the cancer screening test is to determine which patients should be biopsied. In other words, a screening test is a preliminary test. It is not a test to determine who has cancer; instead, it is a test to determine who should be tested further. So the more pragmatic ideal looks like this:

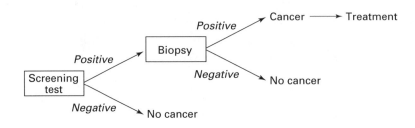

As you may infer from the illustration, a positive screening test can be wrong. That is, a person can be told that his screening test suggests the possibility of cancer, while the biopsy demonstrates that no cancer exists. A positive screening test that is proved wrong is called a false positive. Many call it a "cancer scare."

Can a negative screening test be wrong? The answer is almost certainly yes, although it is very hard to prove. That is because we do not biopsy people with negative screening tests. The only way we ever come to suspect that a negative screening test might have been wrong is when a new cancer becomes clinically obvious soon after a person has a negative test. Recall from the previous chapter the story about my patient's daughter who had metastatic breast cancer diagnosed three months after a normal mammogram. In situations like this, it is reasonable to wonder whether the normal result—or negative screening—was wrong. But as I suggested then, the problem could just as easily be a fast-growing cancer as a falsely negative test. It's impossible to know.

TESTING IN THE REAL WORLD

In the real world, cancer testing is more complex. Test results aren't just positive or negative; often they are somewhere in between. These in-between results may lead to in-between tests: something more thorough than the screening test but a few steps short of a biopsy. Sometimes in-between results lead to a recommendation simply to repeat the screening test after a few months have passed. The reality, therefore, looks more like this:

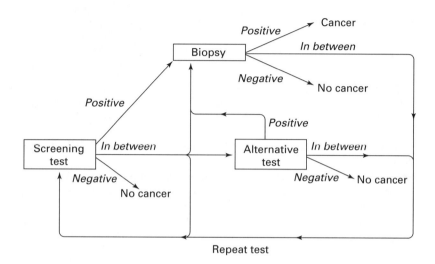

Repeat test

Most people will be on the first negative arrow following a screening test: they will avoid this complex cycle altogether.[2] At the same time, a lot more people will be on the positive or in-between arrows than will ever have cancer. False positive and indeterminate results are inherent features of screening—because unfortunately, we don't have perfect tests.

The woman I told you about at the beginning of this chapter has been on every arrow in this figure, except those leading to a definitive diagnosis. You might think of it as a testing cascade, with one test begetting another. Alternatively, you might think of it as being trapped in an endless cycle, where the patient keeps coming back for more testing. Either way it's no fun. What happened to her may not happen often, but it does happen.

Although the testing process differs depending on which cancer is being sought, some features are common to all cancer testing. The screen-

Table 2   Confirmatory testing for abnormal screening result

Screening test (target cancer)	Early repeat examination[1]	Alternative test[2]	Biopsy
Mammography (breast cancer)	yes	Ultrasound	Needle or excisional biopsy
Fecal occult blood (colon cancer)	not recommended	Barium enema; sigmoidoscopy; colonoscopy	Forceps biopsy during sigmoidoscopy or colonoscopy
PSA blood test (prostate cancer)	yes	Ultrasound	Needle biopsy through rectum
Chest X-ray (lung cancer)	yes	CAT scan	Needle biopsy through chest or during bronchoscopy
Pap smear (cervical cancer)	yes	Colposcopy; test for virus	Forceps biopsy during pelvic exam

[1]Typically the screening test is repeated between three months and six months following the initial abnormal screening test.

[2]See the glossary for a description of each of these tests.

ing test itself is generally the simplest, least disruptive, and safest of all the tests used to detect a cancer. When the screening test is abnormal, confirmatory testing is initiated. The confirmatory testing can range from repeating the screening test earlier than normal (in six months instead of one year, for example) to performing an alternative test that is generally more accurate (and generally more involved) to performing a biopsy (the most definitive test). If the screening test is not too suspicious, an early repeat test or an alternative test is often recommended. But if it is suspicious, a biopsy is generally recommended. The confirmatory testing options for common screening tests are shown in Table 2.

HOW COMMON ARE FALSE POSITIVE TESTS?

Now that you know something about the testing process, I want to give you some sense of how often problems occur. I'll start with the false positive test, or "cancer scare": a positive screening test that, after further confirmatory testing, is determined to be in error. A false positive triggers a process during which people can get hurt, in terms of both their physical and mental health.

The measure of how often a screening test is falsely positive is called a false positive rate: if 100 people are screened and 5 have false positive results, the false positive rate is 5 percent. The false positive rate depends on a number of factors: the test itself, the population being tested, the quality of the testing, and how the test is interpreted. All the common screening tests are plagued by the problem of false positive results.

Mammography

Investigators in Europe have reported false positive rates of about 5 percent for women undergoing mammography for the first time.[3] Women receiving subsequent mammograms were about half as likely to experience a false positive. This is the general pattern with mammography. Here's why: with the first mammogram, the radiologist has no other picture for comparison. All breasts are different, and it is not always clear what is normally different versus what is abnormally different. Without a previous mammogram for reference, therefore, radiologists understandably play it conservative and read more films as abnormal. But with subsequent mammograms there is a point of comparison—an earlier picture of the same breast. Now all the radiologist has to do is look for changes. Something that appeared worrisome in one picture yet is the same in the next becomes a lot less worrisome. So there tend to be fewer false positives on subsequent mammograms.

Investigators at the University of California, San Francisco—who devote particular effort to doing mammography well—report slightly higher false positive rates for first-time exams: about 6 to 7 percent.[4] Following the normal pattern, their subsequent exams then have lower false positive rates. But this is an exceptionally good practice; for the rest of the United States, it appears, the experience is quite different. Some investigators (including myself) have measured what goes on where most patients receive their health care: a typical community practice. Despite the standard mixture of first-time and subsequent testing, the false positive rate for most American women seems to be much closer to 10 percent.[5] The reason? No one knows for sure, but I suspect that most American radiologists err on the side of calling things abnormal (in part, for fear of being sued), which in turn leads to higher false positive rates.

Prostate specific antigen (PSA)

Now let's consider the blood test for prostate cancer, the prostate specific antigen, or PSA. In September 1993, during "Prostate Cancer Awareness Week," a major effort was made to recruit volunteers for testing. Of the more than 30,000 men over age 50 tested in 148 centers, about 3,000 had an abnormally elevated level of PSA; that is, about 10 percent tested positively.[6] Somewhere between a quarter and a third of these men were found to have prostate cancer, making the false positive rate about 7 percent. Others have reported false positive rates in the range of 7 to 11 percent.[7] The most common cause of a false positive PSA is an enlargement of the prostate gland. Because the prostate tends to enlarge with age, PSAs tend to rise with age. Therefore, false positives are less common in younger men and more common in older men.

The false positive rate for subsequent PSA testing depends on whether the initial result was normal or not. If the men with abnormal PSAs are excluded, the false positive rate for a repeat test drops to around 2 percent.[8] In other words, if your test was normal in the past, you are much less likely to have a falsely abnormal test in the future (which in turn means that an abnormal result in subsequent testing is more likely to represent a cancer).[9] However, if your PSA was abnormally elevated once, it is very likely to remain abnormal in the future—even if you never have prostate cancer.

Fecal occult blood testing

Fecal occult blood testing (in which stool is collected and tested for blood as an early sign of colon cancer) has perhaps the highest false positive rate of any screening test, between 8 and 16 percent.[10] The reason is that there are many other possible sources of blood: irritation of the stomach, ulcers in the intestine, and hemorrhoids in the rectum, to name a few. The false positive rate is high enough that many doctors try to prepare patients for a false positive at the time of testing. I tend to say something like, "If your test is positive, it doesn't mean you have cancer—it just means we need to look further and see where the blood is coming from." The false positive rate is about the same on subsequent exams.

Pap smears

It is more difficult to talk about the false positive rate for Pap smears because there are two types of abnormal results. First, roughly 10 percent of Pap smears need to be repeated because of inflammatory changes, generally related to infection. Here, age is again an important variable: adolescents have a false positive rate of more than 15 percent, whereas for women over 60 it is less than 5 percent.[11]

Second, around 5 percent of women undergoing a Pap smear will be told they have a cellular abnormality that is potentially worrisome for cancer. This number also varies by age. Among adolescents the proportion of smears diagnosed with ASCUS (atypical squamous cells of unknown significance) or SIL (squamous intraepithelial lesion) has been reported to be as high as 14 percent. Since almost no women with ASCUS and SIL have or will develop invasive cervical cancer, virtually all of these test results can be considered false positives. However, many of these abnormalities end up being treated, so the problem can also be characterized as unnecessary diagnosis.[12] (Though to be fair, the treatment is fairly simple, often consisting of freezing part of the cervix, much as is done for precancers of the skin.)

So there you have it: our four major screening tests—all of which can, and do, render false positive results. (If you want a rule of thumb for the frequency of false positive cancer tests, put it somewhere between 5 and 10 percent.) In fact, a positive screening test is much more likely to be a false positive than a cancer, generally speaking. So if you receive a worrisome screening test result, just remember: chances are good it is incorrect.

CHANCE OF A FALSE POSITIVE OVER TIME

So far all we have been talking about is the false positive rate after a single screening test, whether it's a first test or a subsequent test. In a program of regular screening, however, you are tested over and over again. Each time you undergo a screening test there's a chance that you will have a cancer scare, that is, that your test will be a false positive. Those are the numbers we've just been looking at. But the chance of you *ever* having this problem accumulates over time. Therefore, the more times you are screened, the more likely you are to have a false positive exam.

To get a sense of the problem, let's do some simple calculations. Imagine a test with a false positive rate of 10 percent for both first-time and subsequent exams. Now consider being tested twice. To determine the chance of having at least one false positive result after two tests, we need to ask the complementary question: What is the chance of *not* having a false positive result after being tested twice? The chance of not having a false positive on an *individual* test is 90 percent (100 percent minus 10 percent). The chance of not having a false positive after *two* tests, therefore, is 90 percent × 90 percent, or 81 percent. So what is your chance of having *at least* one false positive? It is 100 percent minus 81 percent, or 19 percent.

Now let's consider 10 years of annual screening. To determine the chance of having at least one false positive result over this period, we need to follow the same procedure, this time asking what the chance is of *not* receiving a false positive after being tested 10 times. The answer is

$$90\% \times 90\% \times 90\% \times 90\% \times 90\% \times 90\% \times 90\% \times 90\% \times 90\% \times 90\%$$

or

$$0.9^{10} = 0.35 = 35\%$$

Looking then at the complementary situation, we find that the chance of having *at least* one false positive over a 10-year period is 65 percent. In other words, in 10 years of annual screening with this test, you are more likely than not to have at least one cancer scare—and possibly a cascade of additional testing as a result.

Table 3 uses this same approach to demonstrate the effect of five (single-

Table 3   Cumulative risk of one or more false positive tests
in a 10-year program of screening

	Chance of having at least one false positive over ten years when screened:		
False positive rate for an individual test	Every year	Every two years	Every three years
1%	10%	5%	3%
2%	18%	10%	6%
3%	26%	14%	9%
5%	40%	23%	14%
10%	65%	41%	27%

test) false positive rates and three screening frequencies on the chance of having at least one false positive in a 10-year screening program. As this table shows, the cumulative risk of having a cancer scare can be reduced in two ways: have a test with a low false positive rate or test less frequently.

This calculation, though theoretical, is a simple version of the kind of analysis that screening experts do regularly to determine how often to recommend a screening test. The basic trade-off is between missing cancers in between screening tests, on the one hand, and the burden of testing (false positives and subsequent testing), on the other. More frequent screenings mean fewer missed cancers but a higher testing burden. However, the trade-off varies depending on the cancer involved. Analyses of cervical cancer screening, for example, have suggested that Pap smears can be done much less frequently than most women were probably taught (every three years instead of every year) with little, if any, effect on how many cervical cancers are missed. But the change has a big effect on the burden of testing. This kind of analysis is the major reason that most professional organizations recommend that after two or three normal exams, Pap smears be done every three years.[13]

A few studies have tried to measure the cumulative risk of a false positive test. A study at Harvard Pilgrim (a large Boston HMO) looked at women undergoing mammography over a 10-year period.[14] The false positive rate for an individual mammogram (a mix of initial and subsequent exams) was found to be 6.5 percent, which is lower than the average rate in the United States. The typical woman had four mammograms over 10 years, and about a quarter of the women surveyed had at least one false positive exam. The authors stated that, of women who get a mammogram every year for 10 years, 49 percent would be expected to have at least one false positive.[15]

A study in Australia measured additional testing following Pap smear screening.[16] The investigators were specifically interested in the long-term risk of colposcopy, a confirmatory test for an abnormal Pap smear. They estimated that at current rates of testing, the typical 15-year-old girl has a 76.8 percent chance of undergoing a colposcopy sometime in her lifetime. Because virtually all (99 percent) of these exams will not identify a cancer, they conclude that the lifetime risk of a false positive Pap smear is over 75 percent.

These two studies provide us with some perspective about the downsides of testing. If you are a woman who follows screening recommendations for breast and cervical cancer, the chances are better than 50–50 that—at some point in your life—you will have an abnormal test result and will have additional testing recommended. Thus, it is more likely than not that you will spend some time worrying about whether you have breast or cervical cancer. This may not matter much to some, but may to others.

Finally, consider the American randomized trial of fecal occult blood testing discussed in Chapter 1.[17] A third of participants had at least one false positive test over 13 years, and as a consequence all underwent a complete evaluation of their colon (i.e., colonoscopy). A number of doctors wonder if the high false positive rate of fecal occult blood testing is the reason it works—in that it sends many people to have the test that really helps, a colonoscopy.

RISK TO PHYSICAL HEALTH

Do screening tests pose any risks to your physical health? While some may be uncomfortable (mammogram, Pap smear) and others unpleasant (fecal occult blood testing), none of the major screening tests themselves pose a serious physical risk. However, screening tests may start a chain of events in which physical harm is possible. One of the reasons false positive tests are cause for concern, for example, is that before patients learn they don't have cancer they often must undergo tests that pose more serious risks. One of the most common—and one that typically involves sharp tools— is the biopsy.

In the past, a biopsy often involved going to the operating room. It was real surgery involving long incisions using knives. Nowadays, biopsies are increasingly performed in less expensive settings such as doctors' offices, radiology departments, and endoscopy suites. And instead of re- quiring knives, biopsies are performed using needles or forceps (a small jawlike instrument that literally takes a bite of tissue). These less invasive approaches make the process safer and easier, and the patient can usually go home soon afterward.

Nevertheless, complications do occur, and they get worse as biopsies delve deeper inside the body. The complications from a breast or cervix biopsy, for example, are minor compared to the complications from biop- sies of the colon or lung. In the colon, the biopsy procedure involves a long flexible scope that can perforate (poke a hole in) the wall of the colon. If that happens, surgery is needed. Biopsies of the lung occasionally cause the lung to collapse. If that happens, a tube needs to be inserted inside the chest to reexpand the lung. Perforated colons and collapsed lungs are rough even for the young. For the elderly and the debilitated, they can be deadly.

Nevertheless, even these deep biopsies are relatively safe. Perforated colons occur in, at most, one-half of 1 percent of colon biopsies, while col- lapsed lungs occur in about 5 percent of lung biopsies.[18]

That said, it's still no picnic. One of my patients who has a chronically elevated PSA level has undergone multiple prostate biopsies.[19] Let me tell you how they are done. Because the prostate is a long way from the skin— deep in the male pelvis between the penis and the bladder—the easiest way to get a needle into it is through the rectum. A patient lies on his side on an exam table while a condom-covered probe, about the diameter of your thumb, is passed into the rectum (my patient doesn't like this part at all). This probe produces a picture of the prostate using ultrasound (a radar of sorts—the same technique used to take pictures of babies inside pregnant women). The biopsy needle is passed through the probe and into the prostate. Thus the doctor taking the biopsy can view on a small video screen the path of the needle. A prostate biopsy is a relatively safe procedure; only about 1–2 percent of men suffer a major complication requiring hospitalization. Even so, over half will have some sort of complication—generally bloody urine for several days.[20]

My patient—whom I consider an expert in this area—summarizes the process something like this: getting the biopsy is demeaning, and he's uncomfortable for a few days afterward, but it's not the end of the world. After having gone through this four times, though, he's understandably down on the process. When I last asked him about it, he replied: "I'm not dead yet—but what a rat race!"

A DOCTOR BECOMES A PATIENT

While the cancer testing process doesn't pose a great deal of physical risk, it can be pretty uncomfortable and scary. The chairman of radiology at Emory University recently had the misfortune of experiencing firsthand the kinds of problems that can follow a screening test. It is a story best told in his own words, excerpted from a letter published in a radiology journal.[21]

> What is often missing from radiologists' thoughts is firsthand experience with the clinical drama that follows screening or diagnostic tests. My personal anecdote is an example of the clinical aphorism that the only normal patient is one who has not yet been completely worked up.
>
> It began innocently enough with a negative virtual colonoscopy (which involves a CAT scan) that was requested following my routine annual physical examination. Lurking outside the colon were a kidney mass, a 2 cm liver mass and multiple non-calcified nodules in the lungs. Our observant radiologists saw them all.
>
> Further CAT scans of the abdomen demonstrated that the kidney mass was a cyst. The non-enhancing liver lesion was not. A high-resolution lung CAT scan revealed 7–8 non-calcified nodules in the

lower portion of both my lungs. A previous chest X-ray in 1997 was negative.

The CAT scan–guided liver biopsy was not definitive. A PET scan was negative. After much debate, a video-aided thoracoscopy (fiberoptic exam of the lungs) was performed through the ribs. Three small sections of my right lung were removed after the anesthesiologists had collapsed part of it in order to help the surgeons find the nodules. Thorough evaluation by the pathologists made a definitive diagnosis of Histoplasmosis (a common, often asymptomatic, fungal infection).

I awoke in the recovery room after five hours elapsed time with a tube in my chest, a tube in my bladder, a catheter into a vein near my heart, a catheter into an artery in my wrist, a catheter in my spine (for anesthesia), and was being given oxygen in my nose, shots of heparin, a constant infusion of prophylactic antibiotics, and patient-controlled intravenous narcotics.

Over the next four days, the tubes and potent drugs were slowly removed, but the excruciating pain lingered on. However, the nurses were great, the hospital staff superb, the surgeons were the best anywhere and no untoward events or complications occurred. Most of all the outcome was great.

However, it required two weeks at home with Oxycotin and Percodan (narcotic pain killers) before the pain became bearable and a modicum of strength returned. Now five weeks later things are nearly normal except for rib pain caused by the surgical interruption of the nerves. But we are all happy.

He may have been relieved, but he was also motivated to start asking some hard questions about whether radiologists, with remarkably sensitive imaging tests at their disposal, had gotten too far away from what their patients were experiencing. His story certainly makes one wonder whether they are seeing too much.

SENSE OF WELL-BEING

Many people will say that extra testing, the rare risk of physical harm, and the anxiety of false positive and ambiguous results are a small price to pay for early cancer detection. But that really depends on what the benefits of early cancer detection are. If there is a substantial life-expectancy benefit, then the twists and turns of the testing process may indeed be a small price to pay. If, however, there is trivial benefit to early cancer detection—or no benefit at all—it would be best to avoid the process.

How you feel about the trade-off depends on who you are. Different people will feel differently about what constitutes a "substantial" and a "trivial" benefit. Different people will also feel differently about extra testing, false positive results, and ambiguous results, and an individual's attitude may change over time and under different circumstances.

Some people even experience a false positive screening test for cancer in a positive way. At first, of course, they may be very scared; but while they wait for the confirmatory test, they use their time to think about cancer and about what's important in life. And there is a tremendous sense of relief when they are told that they don't have cancer.

The psychological implications of a false positive test have been best studied in mammography. Researchers in Pennsylvania surveyed women who had recently had abnormal mammograms but did not, as things turned out, have cancer.[22] Three months after their false positive, 40 percent of the women were worried about breast cancer—but so were 28 percent of women with normal mammograms. So the researchers asked whether worrying about breast cancer affected the women's moods. About a quarter of women with false positives thought so, as opposed to only 10 percent of women with normal mammograms. In this study at least, then, false positives had some negative psychological aftereffects, but not a great deal.

But it is important to remember that all the women in this study were interviewed at a time when there was no ambiguity: they knew that they did not have cancer. Had they been interviewed at a different time—when they thought they might have cancer—they would perhaps have answered the questions differently.

The degree of negative psychologic impact resulting from false positive tests is likely a function of both how often an individual experiences them and how long the period of ambiguity lasts. It may be a very short period, lasting only a few days (or a few weeks) until a definitive answer is given—and if the answer is good news, as in the Pennsylvania study, that period of ambiguity may seem minor, even beneficial. But for others, definitive answers do not come so quickly, and people may be asked to wait a few months and then repeat the test.

Repeat testing is the most common strategy used following an abnormal Pap smear or an abnormal mammogram. In one study, about 90 percent of women with abnormal mammograms in the Medicare program (women over age 65) had the test repeated. Of these, about half had the repeat test within a month, while most of the rest waited five to seven months.[23] For Pap smears, repeat testing in a few months would be even more common.

For a few patients—the woman with persistently abnormal Pap smears or my patient with a persistently elevated PSA—the ambiguity never ends. The real stressor then becomes uncertainty. These individuals are caught in a seemingly endless cycle of testing: no one has found cancer, but no one can (or will) reassure them that they don't have it. The distressing combination of repeat testing and persistent ambiguity may be enough to push such individuals toward treatment for cancer even though no one has established that cancer is present. Both started the diagnostic process assuming, like most of us, that it could never hurt to look. Now they feel differently: they wonder whether they wouldn't be better off if they'd never been tested in the first place.

SUMMARY

Most of the problems discussed in this chapter are no doubt familiar to you. You probably know people who have had an abnormal screening test—but didn't have cancer. They may have had to undergo multiple tests. They may have even had complications. They probably felt a great deal of relief when it was all over. They may appreciate life more now.

You also may know someone who has suffered from not knowing for sure—someone who has waited, and may still be waiting, for follow-up testing. On this point I am conflicted. I want you to be aware that for some screening tests the best strategy for an abnormal result is to repeat the test after a few months. The downside is obvious: during the waiting period there is ambiguity and, for some, considerable anxiety. At the same time, I believe this "check again later" strategy often is the best way to test for early cancer. As will become clear in later chapters, having information from two points in time may be the key to sorting the wheat (abnormalities that need treatment) from the chaff (abnormalities that are better left alone).

I hope I've given you some sense of how it can hurt to look for cancer. Again, I want to emphasize that just because it can hurt doesn't mean it will. But if you are considering testing, you must understand that false positive tests, with all their consequences—anxiety, potentially endless cycles of testing, and a small risk of physical harm—are side effects of testing. They may even be reason enough for some to choose not to be tested and even forgo a small life-prolonging benefit. Yet despite being the most familiar problems with screening, they are by no means the most important.

THREE   *You may receive unnecessary treatment*

Imagine you had gone through a testing process and had avoided the problems discussed in Chapter 2: false positive tests, repetitive testing, and ambiguous results. Instead the test result was straightforward and clear: you have cancer. At first, you are devastated. You wonder why it had to happen to you. It's as if you've hit the jackpot in some horrible lottery.

On more careful reflection, however, you come to regard the news from a different perspective. Because only people with cancer can benefit from screening, everyone else goes through the testing process for nothing. You are fortunate; you caught the cancer early. Perhaps it can be treated and you will be OK. You may be one of the lucky ones.

The truth, of course, is more complicated. Some people really are lucky: their cancers would have caused problems but were found early and will be cured through treatment. For others, however, the situation is different: their cancers never were going to cause problems. Unfortunately, we can't reliably distinguish between these two groups. Consequently, we treat both.

This is the biggest downside to screening. The problems of false positive tests, repetitive testing, and ambiguous results are dwarfed by the problem of unnecessary diagnosis and treatment.

Let me be clear: when I use the word *unnecessary,* I in no way mean to imply intent. Doctors do not intentionally diagnose cancer unnecessarily, nor do they intentionally treat it unnecessarily. Nevertheless, simply because we cannot distinguish between cancers that do and do not need treatment, people become patients unnecessarily.

And you really do not want to become a cancer patient unnecessarily— not only because receiving a cancer diagnosis can be emotionally devastating, but because unnecessary treatment is harmful to your health. The fact is, many of our cancer treatments are very rough on patients. Surgery, chemotherapy, and radiation all have real side effects, real complications, and a real risk of mortality. No one would want to assume these risks if they knew that their cancer was never going to cause problems.

In this chapter I will argue that we should reconsider how we think about cancer. Not all cancers are the same. Not all cancers spread relentlessly throughout the body. Not all cancers kill people. Instead, the dynamics of cancer are far more heterogeneous: some cancers progress rapidly, some progress slowly, some don't progress at all. And some even regress.

THE EXCEPTIONAL CASE

Most doctors who care for many cancer patients have stories about the very few they thought were terminal but who got better without treatment. The oncologist at our small hospital says he has seen this happen a number of times in his 30 years of practice. In fact, Joe used to collate what he called "remarkable stories" of patients who survived far beyond what was expected. He would share these surprisingly good outcomes with other patients so that they knew not only the average outcome (such as a five-year survival rate) but also what was possible.

One story Joe frequently told concerned a New Hampshire schoolteacher who came to him for care in the mid-1970s. The patient was a middle-aged man whose chest X-ray revealed a large lung cancer. The biopsy showed an unusual type of lung cancer, and an especially deadly one: small cell carcinoma. The prognosis for small cell carcinoma is so poor that researchers measure survival at two years instead of lung cancer's typical five years—and the proportion of patients alive at two years is still less than 30 percent. Because surgery is generally not helpful, Joe started this man on the only treatments available: chemotherapy and radiation.

Chemo and radiation can be hard on patients. In the mid-1970s, moreover, we did not have many of the drugs that now make these treatments more tolerable. The chemo was particularly tough on this patient; he got very sick, and Joe had serious misgivings. As he put it, "I just felt we were beating him up too much." After all, this was a cancer that no one expected to cure, for which the only hope, it was thought, was to slow its progression.

After a lengthy discussion, doctor and patient decided to stop treatment. But Joe continued to see the man every month. Every month he ordered a chest X-ray, and every month the cancer was there. This went on for eight months, with the same cancer appearing unfailingly on the X-ray—no change. Then, in the ninth month, it was gone. It wasn't just smaller: it had disappeared. Some doctors tried to rationalize the change, saying it was a late effect of the treatment. But this did not seem possible: not only did the change occur too long after treatment was discontinued, but it was too dramatic. The patient ascribed the cure to "attitude and appetite." Joe's conclusion was simple: the cancer had regressed all on its own.

This story is exceptional; spontaneous regression of an advanced cancer is exceedingly rare.[1] However, such exceptional cases demonstrate that cancer, even advanced lung cancer, doesn't always do what we expect. Under the right conditions, the human body can turn a cancer around. And if this can happen in large, aggressive cancers, it doesn't seem too great a leap to suppose it would happen even more often in small, early cancers.

CANCER DYNAMICS

In Chapter 1, I presented a simplified model of cancer dynamics. This theoretical model illustrated the preclinical phase of cancer, starting with an abnormal cell and ending when the patient notices symptoms from the cancer. This is the period during which a test might catch a cancer early. I noted that some people have cancers with short preclinical phases (fast-growing cancers), while others have cancers with long preclinical phases (slow-growing cancers). And I pointed out the unfortunate implication of a short preclinical phase: screening tends to miss the fast-growing cancers, the very cancers we would most like to catch.

Thinking about cancer this way has a hidden assumption, which is that all cancers inevitably cause symptoms. Although most people never question this assumption, it has a powerful effect on the way we think about cancer. If all cancers are going to cause problems, then the argument that we should always "do something" about cancer gets stronger, as does the argument that we should definitely look for early forms of cancer (that is, screen for it). But if cancer does not inevitably cause problems, the question of whether to treat it—or even look for it—becomes much more difficult.

Why might a cancer never cause trouble? Consider Figure 3, which uses four arrows to represent four cancers. The arrow labeled "Fast" represents a cancer that is growing fast, one that leads quickly to symptoms and to death. The arrow labeled "Slow" represents a slow-growing cancer, one that leads to symptoms and death but only after many years.

Now let's consider the two cancers that will never cause problems. The arrow labeled "Very slow" represents a cancer that is growing so slowly that it never becomes symptomatic: the person with this cancer will die of some other cause before the cancer even becomes noticeable. As you might guess, this situation is particularly likely with small cancers in the elderly.

The arrow labeled "Nonprogressive" represents a cancer that never causes problems simply because it stops growing or perhaps even shrinks. You may have thought that all cancers progress. That is not the case. Some cancers outgrow their blood supply, and are starved; others are recognized by the host's immune system, and are successfully contained; and some are not aggressive in the first place. In other words, cellular abnormalities can occur that meet the pathologic definition of cancer but never grow—or may even get smaller. These are often referred to as nonprogressive cancers.

Nonprogressive cancers and very slow growing cancers are collectively

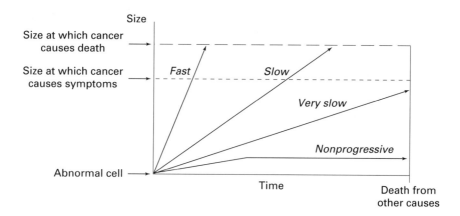

Figure 3.   The spectrum of cancer growth rates.

referred to as pseudodisease (literally, "false disease"). Since the word *disease* implies something that makes, or will make, a person feel sick— something that causes symptoms—pseudodisease is an appropriate word for these asymptomatic cancers.

By definition, therefore, pseudodisease is a type of cancer that need not be treated. In the rest of this chapter, I will share two lines of evidence that demonstrate how pseudodisease can throw a wrench into the works of early cancer detection. The first is based on studies of the dynamics of three cancers—neuroblastoma, renal cell carcinoma, and early breast cancer— each of which can have nonprogressive forms. The second is based on our national experience with prostate cancer in the last quarter of the twentieth century and the finding that many more people have prostate cancer than will ever experience symptoms of it—much less die of it. Both these lines of evidence have an important upshot: we find much more cancer than can possibly matter to patients.

SOME CANCERS DON'T PROGRESS

The natural dynamics of how various cancers grow (or don't grow) is not well studied in humans. The reason is obvious: we rarely watch something a pathologist calls "cancer"; instead we cut it out, radiate it, or try to kill it with drugs. Nevertheless, a few dynamic observations of untreated cancers have been made which confirm that not all cancers progress and that pseudodisease exists.

Neuroblastoma

Perhaps the best observations about the dynamics of untreated cancer come from studies of neuroblastoma, a rare form of cancer that typically affects young children.[2] These cancers, which generally start near the kidney, make adrenaline-like substances. They can get as large as a grapefruit (which in an infant is huge), can invade major blood vessels (like the aorta), and can metastasize to major organs (like the liver). They can kill children.

Japanese health authorities, recognizing the seriousness of this cancer, started an aggressive, nationwide neuroblastoma screening program in 1985.[3] With the goal of catching the cancer early, they screened infants at six months, employing a relatively simple test: urine analysis for the breakdown products of adrenaline. Once the search for neuroblastoma began, the Japanese authorities found more of it. The total number of children diagnosed with the disease more than doubled, and in the group being screened—children less than one year of age—it increased almost fivefold.

Some Japanese physicians found this trend very concerning.[4] They worried that the new cancers being found in infants were not the ones that would go on to kill older children. And they worried about the dangers of treatment for neuroblastoma (surgery and chemotherapy), which could also kill children. To address these concerns, one group of pediatric oncologists decided to watch infants with small cancers (smaller than a tennis ball) that were not obviously doing damage: that is, they had not invaded major vessels, and were not producing a large amount of adrenaline-like substances.[5]

Of 25 six-month-old infants being treated by this group of doctors for neuroblastoma, 17 had cancers that met these criteria. The parents of 11 of those infants chose not to have their child operated on or receive chemotherapy but instead to have them watched carefully, with a monthly ultrasound and urine test. This decision turned out to be a good one: 10 of the 11 cancers began to get smaller right away. The other continued to grow until the child reached one year of age and then it, too, began to regress. Thus, all 11 infants had pseudodisease. The authors concluded that the right strategy for neuroblastoma meeting these criteria is not treatment, but careful observation to determine which way the cancer is going—a strategy known as "watchful waiting."

More recent research has raised the question of whether pseudodisease is so common in neuroblastoma that even looking for the cancer does children more harm than good. I will describe those findings in the next chapter.

Kidney cancer

We often stumble on renal cell carcinoma (kidney cancer) by accident. The typical scenario goes something like this: a patient has a CAT scan or ultrasound of the abdomen for some complaint about digestion—a symptom having nothing to do with the kidney. But surprise, a small mass is found on the kidney. Now, it turns out that a kidney biopsy is neither easy nor particularly reliable. And even though we have two kidneys, no one is in a rush to remove a well-functioning one. Instead of biopsying or removing the organ, therefore, some doctors and patients have opted for a different approach: periodically (every six months or so) rescanning the kidney to determine whether the mass is growing.

Radiologists at New York University Medical Center reported on following—in a few cases for up to eight years—the growth of 40 small kidney tumors (defined as less than 3.5 cm, or 1.4 inches, in diameter).[6] The three fastest-growing tumors increased in diameter only about 1 cm per year (about one-third of an inch). The remaining 37 grew considerably more slowly: less than 0.6 cm (0.25 inch) per year. Some didn't grow at all. Twenty-six of the tumors grew big enough that they were ultimately removed, but fourteen never grew large enough for the doctors to recommend surgery. More important, no one died of renal cell carcinoma, and no one developed metastases or any symptoms from their cancer.

This study is another example showing how we may need to rethink our approach to early cancer treatment. Each patient was carefully followed over time so that the doctors could learn about the dynamics of that particular cancer. Those who had cancers that were really growing had their kidney removed, those with indolent cancers were spared the operation. Small kidney cancers provide another instance in which pseudodisease is common and where watchful waiting can be superior to immediate treatment.

Breast cancer

The early form of breast cancer that we most frequently detect with mammography is ductal carcinoma in situ, or DCIS. This cancer is confined within a single duct—one of the many small tubes that transport milk from the glands in the breast to the nipple. Because the idea of simply "watching" a small breast cancer is sacrilegious in our current clinical culture, DCIS is almost always treated (with mastectomy, lumpectomy, or radiation). We therefore know very little about the dynamics of this emotionally charged cancer.

Some insight can be gained from two sets of observations. The first involves women whose DCIS was missed at the time of biopsy. These cases were found by reviewing thousands of breast biopsies from the 1950s and 1960s in Nashville, Tennessee, and Bologna, Italy, that were reported as benign and, as a result, not treated.[7] Thus they provide important information about the risk of developing invasive breast cancer for women with DCIS. In the Tennessee study, 25 percent (7 of 28) of women developed invasive breast cancer within 10 years of being biopsied; the Italian rate was 11 percent (3 of 28) within 20 years. Looking at these numbers another way, we can say that 75 percent and 89 percent of the women, respectively, did *not* develop invasive breast cancer: that is, they had pseudodisease. A third study of women treated only with excisional biopsy reported similar findings: 90 percent did not go on to develop breast cancer within the next 10 years.[8] From these data we learn two things: most women with DCIS do not develop invasive breast cancer, and for those who do progress to cancer, the process is slow—slow enough that watchful waiting might make sense.[9]

The second set of observations concerns how long women with DCIS live. In a study using nationwide data, researchers in San Francisco examined the life expectancy of women with breast cancer (most of whom were treated for the disease) compared to other women of similar age.[10] Not surprisingly, women with metastatic breast cancer were 12 times more likely to die than similar-aged women. For women with early-stage invasive breast cancer, the likelihood dropped to twice as high. Women with DCIS, however, were 20 to 30 percent *less* likely to die than similar-aged women.

This curious finding is the product of an interplay of two factors. Most women diagnosed with DCIS are women who have had mammograms and, as a group, are healthier than average. But don't miss the big picture here. What is astounding is that the diagnosis of DCIS does not have the obvious adverse impact on life expectancy that we generally associate with the word *cancer*. An ardent proponent of medical care might argue that the nondeleterious effect of DCIS on life expectancy means our treatment of DCIS is really, really good. But there is a more realistic—and less flattering—explanation: most DCIS is pseudodisease. Although rarely done, watchful waiting may be a reasonable strategy for many women with DCIS as well.

THERE IS MORE CANCER THAN CAN POSSIBLY MATTER

How hard we look affects how much prostate cancer we find

The most compelling evidence that pseudodisease is a real problem comes from our national experience with prostate cancer. Prostate cancer is a pretty common form of cancer. In fact, more men will be diagnosed with prostate cancer than any other form of cancer, excluding only skin cancer. And about 3 percent of men will die from the disease. But the question of exactly how many men have this cancer depends on how hard you look.

I first became aware of this problem after reviewing a study that had nothing to do with prostate cancer; rather, it was about how best to treat urinary difficulties in older men.[11] The 556 men all had enlarged prostates that were making it difficult for them to empty their bladder.[12] Half of the men got immediate surgery; the other half were carefully followed and offered surgery if they got worse (one-quarter of this group ultimately had surgery). The study was a randomized trial, meaning that the decision to treat surgically was made essentially by the flip of a coin. In other words, the two groups of men were more or less identical—at least at the outset. Once treatment started, however, the surgery group developed a lot more cancer: 24 cases after three years, as opposed to only 8 in the group that did not get immediate surgery (7 of which were diagnosed only because the patients had the surgery at a later date). So if one were to consider the treatment actually received, the count would be 31 cancers among those undergoing surgery versus only 1 among those not undergoing surgery.

Does prostate surgery cause prostate cancer? Of course not. But it does find it. To understand why, you have to know a little bit about the surgery, which is known as transurethral resection of the prostate—TURP for short. Its purpose is to remove some of the prostate, thus creating a larger passageway for urine to flow out. In practice, this involves putting an instrument through the penis and shaving off small pieces of prostate from the inside. As is the case for all tissue removed from the body during an operation, these shavings (typically 15 to 30 pieces) are sent to the pathology department. The pathologists then look carefully at the tissue under the microscope. And they find cancers. Most of these cancers, however, would never have been found were it not for the operation.

Transurethral resection of the prostate was quite popular in the late 1970s and 1980s and was performed frequently enough that the reported cases of prostate cancer began to rise. Then, in the late 1980s, a new way to find prostate cancer was developed: a blood test that measured prostate specific antigen (PSA). This test caused the number of cancer cases to skyrocket. Figure 4 shows how these two procedures affected the number of new cases of prostate cancer as reported to the U.S. government's Surveillance Epidemiology and End Results (SEER) program.[13]

I don't know of any cancer researcher who argues that this graph reflects some change in the true occurrence of prostate cancer. The changes are too big, they occur too fast, and they go up and down (and up again).[14] What it does reflect is the changing practice style of physicians: we are

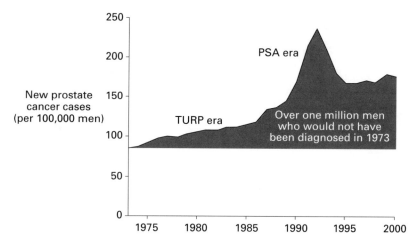

Figure 4. Prostate cancer in the United States, 1973–2000: new cases.

looking much harder for prostate cancer now—and finding it more often. The net effect of TURP and PSA testing is astounding: over the last quarter century more than a million men have been diagnosed with prostate cancer who would not have received this diagnosis in the early 1970s.

But finding more may not be a good thing

Is finding these early cancers a good thing or a bad thing? It could be either. The efficacy of prostate cancer screening has not yet been tested with the best scientific method, a randomized trial, so we can only guess.[15] We do know screening has an effect: the dramatic rise in the number of new cases of prostate cancer in the last quarter century is proof enough. Yet one would like to see a corresponding reduction in the number of prostate cancer deaths. Although such a reduction, by itself, wouldn't prove that prostate cancer screening worked (it could be that the *treatment* of advanced prostate cancer has improved over time), one would certainly be more sanguine about screening if the death rate from prostate cancer was clearly falling.

But it's not. The SEER database also tracks the number of people who

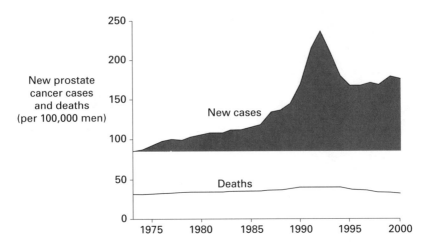

Figure 5.   Prostate cancer in the United States, 1973–2000: new cases and deaths.

die from prostate cancer. Figure 5 presents this information along with the number of new cases. Take a look at the lower line, which indicates the death rate. Although it moves up and down a tiny bit, as you can see, the prostate cancer mortality rate hasn't changed much since 1973. It increased a little from the mid-1970s to the early 1990s and has been falling the last few years. Some have argued that the recent decline attests to the usefulness of testing for prostate cancer, but it could just as easily reflect better treatment. In any case, the big picture is that over a million more men were diagnosed with prostate cancer in the last quarter century, but there has been little change in the number of deaths.

In considering these data, I am reminded of one of the cardiologists who trained me at the Salt Lake City VA. I was a resident working 26-hour shifts in the intensive care unit. He would arrive every morning at 5:30 to see the patients he and I were responsible for. Sometimes a patient—one with a failing heart, perhaps, or having difficulty breathing—was not doing well. He would examine the patient and the charts that illustrated the physiologic trends of the preceding hours. Then he'd look me in the eye and announce, "What you are doing is not working. It's time to try something different." No beating around the bush. The bluntness hurt a bit, but I always respected his forthright assessment. And it is time for a forthright assessment with regard to prostate cancer: what we are doing is not working. Because in the final analysis, most of these one million extra cases of prostate cancer represent nothing more than pseudodisease: disease that would never progress far enough to cause symptoms—or flat-out would never progress at all.

But what, you might ask, is the harm in finding all this pseudodisease? Simply put: unnecessary treatment. Most of the million men whose prostate cancer is found because of superior screening have to undergo some sort of treatment, whether radical surgery or radiation. A few (less than 1 percent) die from surgery, but many experience significant complications: 17 percent need additional treatment because they have difficulty urinating following surgery; 28 percent must wear pads because they have the opposite problem—they cannot hold their urine; and more than half are bothered by a loss of sexual function (inability to have an erection). Among men undergoing radiation, 19 percent still suffer from radiation damage to the rectum two months afterward, and over a third report diarrhea or bowel urgency as much as two years later.[16]

You should know that many doctors are concerned about this problem. There is probably no cancer in which the existence of pseudodisease is more widely accepted and the value of early detection more vigorously questioned. Whether to treat early prostate cancers is a topic of open discussion between doctors and patients. Many older men with small cancers now opt for watchful waiting rather than undergoing an operation, radiation, or chemotherapy. And there is accumulating evidence that this conservative approach makes sense. One Connecticut study found that men with low-grade prostate cancer who chose watchful waiting had the same life span as similar-aged men who did not have prostate cancer.[17]

I should be clear that none of this should be interpreted as saying that PSA testing will never work. In fact, while many men may have been hurt by the ensuing treatment, a few others may have been helped. And it is possible that the PSA test can be modified such that it finds much less cancer and therefore makes much more sense.[18] But right now we need to be clear about the primary effect of the way it has been used so far: it has been making men sick.

And there is yet more to find

Doctors have a saying about prostate cancer: more men die *with* it than *from* it. Another way of putting it is that, for prostate cancer, there is more pseudodisease than real disease. How did we get into this predicament? The answer is simple: by testing for cancer.

Prostate cancer is certainly the most dramatic example of how early detection efforts can go awry. Although you might think that we are finding all the prostate cancer we possibly can, evidence shows that this is not the case. The evidence in question comes from studies in which pathologists—doctors who specialize in examining human tissue under the microscope—examine the prostates of people not known to have cancer. (Pathologists only get this opportunity after people die—as part of an autopsy—or when surgeons remove the entire prostate for some reason other than prostate cancer.) In a number of studies, prostate glands have been collected at autopsy and examined systematically for cancer.[19] The prevalence of cancer in these studies ranges from 13 to 37 percent; in other words, as many as a third of all men (a mixture of young and old) seem to have prostate cancer. Pathologists at the Cleveland Clinic took another approach, examining the prostate glands removed during operations for bladder cancer.[20] They found that 33 of the 72 patients— close to half—had unsuspected prostate cancer. Among men over age 60, the proportion was higher still: almost 60 percent.[21]

If somewhere around half of older men have prostate cancer and only about 3 percent die of it, the potential for unnecessary diagnosis and treatment is huge. And how does this problem get worse? When doctors (and patients) try to find more small, early cancers.

SUMMARY

Not all cancers should be treated. Some small cellular abnormalities that are called "cancer" will not progress to cause symptoms or death. Others will progress so slowly that people will die of something else before they ever have symptoms of cancer. In each case, the cancers are best considered pseudodisease. Pseudodisease is a particular problem for the elderly, who are at the highest risk of dying from something other than cancer. But as I have shown, it can also be a problem for the young (such as women with DCIS) and very young (infants with neuroblastoma). And for pseudodisease, treatment *is* worse than the disease: the only thing it can do is hurt people.

That said, however, it is practically impossible to know for sure whether an individual cancer is, in fact, pseudodisease. The only way we know pseudodisease exists is from observations made on groups of individuals. We know that some cancers, such as neuroblastoma, renal cell carcinoma, and early breast cancer, actually regress. And we know that many more men have prostate cancer than will ever experience symptoms from it, much less die of it. We can infer some ballpark probabilities about the chance that an early cancer is pseudodisease—somewhere between 50 and 80 percent of DCIS and screen-detected prostate cancers, for example, are pseudodisease—but we can't say just which ones. And there is no denying that every type of cancer discussed in this chapter has the potential to kill.

The fact that pseudodisease exists suggests that the correct approach to cancer is not always treatment. Instead, watchful waiting may be a reasonable strategy for many early cancers, giving doctors time to sort out which cancers truly need treatment. The prospect of confusion (and anxiety) about how best to deal with pseudodisease, moreover, may lead some to consider another approach: a more cautious attitude toward testing in general. Because looking hard for cancer only escalates the risk of having to confront pseudodisease—as will become clear in the next chapter.

FOUR

You may find a cancer
you would rather not know about

You are probably beginning to appreciate that the diagnosis of "cancer" can have widely different implications. Testing healthy people identifies a spectrum of cancer: while some are destined to cause symptoms, others are not. Unfortunately, it is practically impossible to be certain which is which by looking at a collection of cells under the microscope. So doctors aren't sure about which cancers should be treated.

What we are sure about is that the way to avoid this dilemma is not to be tested for cancer in the first place. If you are never tested, you will never have to worry about pseudodisease—those cancers that don't progress to cause symptoms. Most of us, however, will consider some cancer screening at some point in our lives. Many will also be evaluated for medical problems unrelated to cancer, which may involve diagnostic tests that, while appropriate to the problem, are also capable of detecting early cancers. Understanding the chance of finding pseudodisease may help you decide when to be screened and what to do if a cancer is found unexpectedly.

Testing and pseudodisease go hand in hand. In the last chapter I focused on the fact that not all cancers progress, therefore not all cancers need treatment. In this chapter, I will discuss a related concept: that there is a lot of cancer that can be found, which means that testing can find too many cancers. The prostate cancer example discussed in Chapter 3 illustrates this more general problem: the harder we look for any type of cancer, the more we find. And the more we find, the more likely it is that what we find is pseudodisease. In other words, one downside of testing is that you might find a cancer you would rather not know about.

FINDING THE UNEXPECTED

About five years ago one of my patients called me because he was hoarse. Indeed, I barely recognized his voice on the phone. I asked him whether he had been sick. He said no; he felt fine, nothing bothered him beside the hoarseness. I asked him how long he had been hoarse. He said about six weeks.

That got me worried. The duration of hoarseness and the lack of other symptoms made laryngitis or some other upper respiratory infection unlikely. And although he had quit about three years earlier, he had been a long-term smoker. These two facts made me worry about cancer, either of the vocal cords or of the lung.[1]

One of the nice things about a small hospital is that the doctors are able to connect with one another pretty easily. It just so happens that the ENT (ear, nose, and throat) doctor is down the hall from me, so I walked to his office, told him about my patient, and asked if he would look at his vocal cords for me. He agreed and made an appointment to see the patient. When he performed the examination a few days later, he found a small tumor, which he biopsied. It was cancer.

However, it was an early cancer. It hadn't spread, and most of it came out during the biopsy itself. The patient's hoarseness resolved itself almost immediately. He was given a short course of radiation and told to come back if he got hoarse again. That would have been the end of it—except someone along the way had also ordered a chest X-ray.

Now, some doctors might argue that he should have had a chest X-ray anyway, given the possibility of lung cancer. I would counter that once we found the cancer responsible for the hoarseness we did not need to go looking for a second cancer. But the horse was out of the barn. Although the lungs looked fine, the radiologist expressed some concern about a possible widening of the mediastinum (the region between the lungs), which could represent a second cancer. And so the radiologist suggested a CAT scan of the chest.

The CAT scan was normal. The radiologist affirmed that the mediastinum was fine and that the chest X-ray had been misleading. But the CAT scan had gone well below the chest, to include organs in the abdomen: the liver, stomach, and kidneys.[2] And on the right kidney there was a mass about the size of a golf ball. It was almost certainly cancer.

So a patient calls complaining of hoarseness and gets diagnosed with kidney cancer. One has absolutely nothing to do with the other; it was just dumb luck.[3]

I've told this story at a number of physician gatherings in the past few years, and I always get the same response: laughter. That doesn't mean they are uncaring or enjoy hearing about the misfortune of others. Instead, the laughter is because most have experienced similar episodes and are familiar with the resulting quandary: is this a lethal cancer or an innocuous one? Should I recommend the kidney be removed or that it be watched?

Almost all doctors have had the experience of stumbling onto a cancer that has nothing to do with the patient's initial complaint. Most have the sense of feeling trapped by the finding and compelled to act. But many also wonder if their action won't create as many problems as it solves and whether the patient might not have been better off without having been tested.

THE HARDER WE LOOK, THE MORE WE FIND

Most people, when they hear that a doctor has unexpectedly found a cancer, feel genuine concern and empathy for the patient. Their next reaction is equally understandable: to remind the patient that he is lucky the doctor found it when she did. The assumption here is that the cancer would ultimately grow and cause problems. But as we have seen, that may not be the case. Some people have cancer and never know it: they never develop symptoms, and they die from some other cause.

Whether or not a cancer is found is a function, in part, of its size. Big cancers are easier to find than small cancers. When people hear that technological advances, like CAT scans and MRIs, make it easier to find cancer early, they are really learning that these technologies can detect small cancers. Without these technologies, many small cancers would go unnoticed. Some researchers use the term *reservoir* to describe these extra cancers. I like this description because it conveys the idea that more cancer exists than is obvious on the surface. To explore this idea, let us begin by considering how an enhanced ability to see cancer affects who gets diagnosed.

Imagine testing 40 people with a relatively crude test—one that can detect only large abnormalities. A good example is the physical exam performed by a doctor, which might reliably detect a softball-sized cancer in the abdomen.[4] Let us assume that one of the 40 people has one of these large cancers. The situation might be illustrated like this:

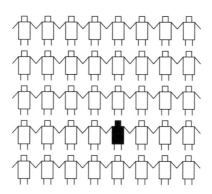

Now, imagine a test better able to detect small abnormalities—a CAT scan, for example, capable of detecting a golf ball–sized cancer. This time, among the 40 people tested, let us assume five cancers are found: four that are golf ball–sized and one that is softball-sized:

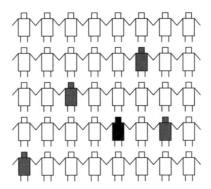

New and "better" tests—meaning more sensitive, better able to detect smaller and smaller abnormalities—will of course be developed in the future. Imagine a *hyper* scan that can reliably detect cancer the size of a pea (something we are pretty close to now). A lot of people have these small cancers. If all 40 people are tested again, let us say 15 cancers are found: 10 that are pea-sized, four that are golf ball–sized, and one that is softball-sized:

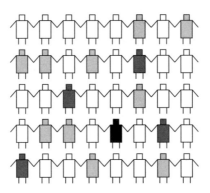

So the answer to the question of who has cancer depends in part on how hard we look. As long as there is a reservoir of undetected cancer, the harder we look, the more we will find. And as we find more, more of what we find will be small abnormalities—the very abnormalities that are most likely to be pseudodisease.

MORE IMAGING, MORE KIDNEY AND LUNG CANCER

Today, increasingly, we find cancer using sophisticated diagnostic technologies: ultrasounds, CAT scans, and MRIs. (Because each of these machines ultimately produces a picture, their use is collectively referred to as imaging.) Because they find more than we ever thought possible, these imaging technologies are changing our picture of certain cancers, particularly cancers of the kidney and the lung.

Kidney cancer

Most doctors think of renal cell carcinoma (kidney cancer) as a pretty rare cancer. But when a group of Canadian executives were screened in the mid-1990s using abdominal ultrasound (not a particularly sensitive test), renal cell carcinoma was found to be quite prevalent—much more so than in the general population.[5] While it is possible that executives are at higher risk for this cancer, it is also possible that there is simply more renal cell carcinoma out there than we think—and that it doesn't tend to be found because no one is actively looking for it.

Other researchers have carefully examined the kidneys of patients who have end-stage renal failure (either they have received a kidney transplant or are undergoing dialysis) using a combination of ultrasound, CAT scans, and needle biopsy.[6] They report finding renal cell carcinoma at stunningly high rates: 40 and 100 times more frequently than in the general population.[7] While it is quite possible that people with kidney failure are at higher risk for this cancer, it is exceedingly unlikely that the increased risk is this big.[8] I suspect what is really happening is that patients with renal failure simply have more systematic examinations of their kidneys than do normal healthy people. In other words, doctors are looking harder and discovering a considerable reservoir of undiagnosed renal cell carcinoma.

Lung cancer

As I mentioned earlier, no professional organization currently recommends screening for lung cancer. But there are certainly good reasons to think hard about lung cancer screening: it is the cancer responsible for the most years of life lost; our treatment for patients with symptomatic disease is pretty ineffective; and it is easy to identify a high-risk group to screen—smokers. In fact, I cannot think of a cancer for which a stronger case could be made for carefully considering the benefits of screening. Nevertheless, as we think about looking harder at people's lungs, it is worth reviewing what others have found in the past.

The late 1970s and early 1980s saw a flurry of interest in chest X-ray screening for lung cancer. The major American study in this area was done at the Mayo clinic, a randomized trial involving more than 9,000 male smokers.[9] Half had routine chest X-rays every four months; half did not have routine chest X-rays and would only have a chest X-ray if there were symptoms of lung cancer. Not surprisingly, more lung cancer was found in the first group—206 cases over six years, versus only 160 cases in the control group.

These "extra" 46 cases have been the source of considerable debate.[10] Remember, it was a randomized trial: the men agreed to be assigned to one group or the other solely by chance. This process is the best way to ensure that the groups are similar at the start of the study and that any subsequent differences observed are the result of whatever intervention they are subjected to. Since the same number of people died from lung cancer in each group, the authors concluded that chest X-ray screening did not save lives. The X-ray group, however, did have 29 percent more cases of diagnosed lung cancer. Then again, recent long-term follow-up showed that some of the people with lung cancer in the X-ray group lived another 15 or 20 years—much longer than expected for a patient with lung cancer—raising questions about whether they really had what we usually think of as lung cancer. Could it be that by looking harder, the radiologists were finding cases of lung cancer that would never have progressed? Could there be pseudodisease in lung cancer?

For lung cancer, just about our most feared malignancy, this is a pretty radical idea. But it is an idea we must confront given the most recent testing strategy for lung cancer: spiral CAT scanning. Although computer-assisted tomography (CAT) scans have been around for some 30 years, until recently they have been too slow to image the lungs; patients needed to breathe during the scan, which blurred the image. Spiral CAT scanners, however, are fast enough to scan the lungs while a patient holds his breath. This technological advance has the potential to detect a lot of pseudodisease in the lung.

One of the first reports on mass screening using spiral CAT scans was from Japan.[11] A mobile unit was driven around the city of Matsumoto, five neighboring towns, and 23 nearby villages and ultimately scanned about 4,000 volunteers. Nineteen had lung cancer. That may not sound like much, but it was almost 10 times the number found in an earlier mass screening program with chest X-rays in the same area. And there was another surprising result: roughly equivalent numbers of lung cancers were found in smokers as in nonsmokers.

This finding is counter to everything doctors have ever learned about lung cancer. Our clinical experience is that lung cancer is almost always deadly. We also know that smokers are at least 10 times more likely to die of lung cancer than nonsmokers. Not only that, but smokers are also 10 times as likely to develop clinical lung cancer—that is, to seek medical care because of symptoms from lung cancer. The fact that as many cancers might be found in nonsmokers as in smokers means that we can overdiagnose lung cancer—and in the Matsumoto case, apparently did: at least for the nonsmokers. Again this is a case of pseudodisease: physicians looking so hard that they find lung cancers that will never affect their patients.

MORE BIOPSIES, MORE PROSTATE CANCER

The general relationship between how hard doctors look and how much cancer is found also applies to biopsies: the more tissue examined, the more likely it is that malignancy will turn up. This phenomenon is particularly important whenever doctors are looking for a cancer that cannot be felt or seen. The current clinical setting where this is most likely to occur is in the detection of prostate cancer.

The problem arises when urologists (specialists in the male urinary and sex organs) are looking for prostate cancer in men with elevated PSA—prostate specific antigen. As described in Chapter 3, in large part because of this blood test almost a million additional men have been diagnosed with prostate cancer in the last 25 years. Consider a typical scenario. A patient has an elevated PSA level, but the doctor cannot feel a lump on the prostate. Because there is no obvious place to biopsy, the urologist takes six biopsies, each one involving a separate insertion of a needle, to search for cancer in various parts of the prostate. The goal is to sample throughout the prostate, with three biopsies on each side: one at the top, one at the mid portion, and one at the base. But no matter how systematic the approach, it still boils down to extracting six samples, each the size of a wood splinter, from an organ the size of a golf ball.

Numbers are useful here. The volume of the typical prostate is 30,000 cubic millimeters.[12] The six biopsy specimens typically represent about 150 cubic millimeters—roughly one-half of 1 percent of the organ. And because only part of each specimen is sliced and placed on a glass slide, the volume of tissue actually examined by the pathologist is about 3 cubic millimeters (or 1/10,000 of the gland). The examination of the slide then proceeds in stages: first the slides are assessed with the naked eye; then the entire slide is viewed using low-power magnification (20 times larger than life). Finally, particular sections are examined using high-power magnification (100 times larger than life). Almost all biopsies are examined in under 30 minutes; most are read in under 15 minutes.

You might be thinking that a number of variables here could influence the chance of a prostate cancer diagnosis in an individual. More needle biopsy specimens—more cancer. More specimen slices placed on glass slides—more cancer. More time spent examining tissue—more cancer.

While all this is true, I think the first variable is most important. And the doctors performing the biopsies are also beginning to appreciate how the number of biopsies might matter. Researchers at Ohio State University recently reported on 74 patients who underwent prostate biopsies using a new strategy involving 12 needle biopsies—*double* the usual number.[13] Over half—40 patients—were found to have prostate cancer. Thirty of these were identified in one of the six biopsy specimens used in the conventional approach. The other 10 were diagnosed based on the extra six specimens. So the additional biopsies found more cancer.

Researchers in Canada went a step further.[14] They examined 37 men with worrisome PSA levels in whom doctors had been unable to find prostate cancer. (And it wasn't for a lack of trying: to be in this study, men had to have had *at least* three prior biopsy procedures, each one involving six to eight needle biopsies.) The technique they used, "saturation biopsy," involved taking between 32 and 38 needle biopsies of the prostate. Although others had looked for and not found cancer at least three separate times, these researchers found another five cases. Look harder—more cancer.

BETTER SAFE THAN SORRY?

At this point you might be thinking, "Isn't it a good thing to find more cancer? I understand that some of these cancers might not progress, but some might. Isn't it better to be safe than sorry?"

It is a good question. But which course of action is really "safer" and which is more likely to lead one to be "sorry" is not immediately clear. So the question is really more about balancing risks. A better way of putting it might therefore be: "Are the risks of inaction greater than the risks of treatment?"

How you answer depends on a number of factors: the likelihood of those extra cancers causing problems, the extent to which early treatment will change the course of those cancers destined to cause problems, and the degree of harm that treatment can cause. Your own personal values also matter tremendously. How would you feel if you missed a chance to do something about an early cancer? And how would you feel about being made to worry unnecessarily about cancer or about receiving treatment unnecessarily? These are not easy questions to answer.

The treatments for kidney, lung, and prostate cancer should not be taken lightly. Definitive treatment involves surgery. Although deaths following prostate removal are rare (less than 1 percent die from operations), they are more common following kidney removal (about 2 percent) and lung removal (5 percent following partial lung removal, over 10 percent following total lung removal).[15] Complications from surgery, however, are not at all uncommon. All surgeries increase the risk of heart attack, stroke, and blood clots; lung removal puts patients at higher risk to contract pneumonia; and prostate removal often affects men's urinary and sexual function. Chemotherapy and radiation treatments pose additional risks.

So are the risks of inaction always greater than the risks of treatment? Consider the extreme case: let's say that a large population of healthy people is tested monthly with *hyper* scans and some evidence of kidney, lung, and prostate cancer is found in 90 percent of them. Since so much disease is found and we know that only a small fraction will ever lead to symptoms (much less death), we must conclude that almost all of what was found must be pseudodisease. Given this scenario and the risks of treatment, I suspect you would argue that inaction is preferable to treatment.

How about the opposite extreme: in an exceptionally well targeted screening program (testing only high-risk persons with a test that is not excessively sensitive), very few cancers are found, 90 percent of which are destined to cause real problems. Now you might be willing to take on the risk of treatment (assuming it works), accepting that 10 percent of the time it would be unnecessary.

Of course, the reality is somewhere in between, but I hope that thinking about the extremes helps convey a general principle: the more cancer that is detected, the more likely it is that pseudodisease is being found and the more likely that the risks of treatment are greater than the risks of inaction.

This whole balancing act can be disconcerting. Once an early cancer is found, a patient is faced with a bewildering array of decisions—any one of which might lead to regret. No one wants to unnecessarily face the anxiety associated with a diagnosis of a potentially fatal disease. So the answer to the question "Isn't it a good thing to find cancer?" may not always be yes. In fact, there may be times when it is better not to look.

MORE HARM THAN GOOD?
THE CASE OF NEUROBLASTOMA

In the last chapter I described a rare form of cancer called neuroblastoma. A childhood cancer that typically starts near the kidney, it may metastasize to major organs and lead to death, but it also may spontaneously regress without any treatment. Consequently, some doctors advise that children with small cancers be watched instead of being subjected to immediate surgery.

But if your child had a neuroblastoma, wouldn't you want to know? Then doctors could at least watch it, and if the cancer became aggressive they could act quickly. Surprisingly, the answer is probably no. Two large studies suggest that you don't even want to look for this cancer—at least not given the current state of medical practice.

One of the studies was conducted in the Canadian province of Quebec, the other in six states of Germany.[16] All together almost two million young children were screened using a simple urine test. These screened children were then compared to children in the general population—children who did not get screened. In each study, screening turned up about twice as many cases of neuroblastoma as expected.[17] But in neither case did finding this extra disease appear to help: there was no difference between screened and unscreened children in terms of the death rate from this cancer. In fact, in both studies, the death rate was actually a tiny bit higher among screened children. Apparently screening found the cancers that did not need treatment and did not change the course of those that did. Both studies concluded that screening for neuroblastoma does no good.

But I doubt most would think that was a sufficient summary of what happened—not if you know the whole story. Although screening rendered no obvious benefit, there *were* obvious harms. Twice as many children as expected were diagnosed with the disease (investigators from the German study estimated that 99 out of 149 were diagnosed unnecessarily). It seems reasonable to surmise that lots of parents worried unnecessarily about their child having cancer. More significant, though, are the complications that ensued from treatment of the disease. In the German study, three of the 149 children diagnosed with neuroblastoma died, one from complications of chemotherapy, and two following surgery. The Canadian study reported that although all 44 children with screen-detected cancer were alive six years later, the treatment was not problem-free. One child developed leukemia because of the chemotherapy he received for neuroblastoma; this required a bone marrow transplant. He then suffered a transplant complication: graft versus host disease, a painful reaction in which the new marrow attacks the body of the transplant recipient. Another child developed intestinal blockage because of the surgery she received for neuroblastoma. Since then she has required more surgery, has had more complications, and she is now in a persistent vegetative state.

Some might argue this is a drop in the bucket of the two million children screened. But I think these five children provide a good reason not to look for neuroblastoma at all. The fact is, it's hard for doctors (and parents) not to treat something called cancer. And treatment can hurt.

HOW MUCH MORE CANCER IS THERE TO FIND?

The problem I have been describing happens because there is an underlying reservoir of cancer that doctors would never know about unless they looked. The larger this reservoir, the more cancer there is to be found. Some pathologists have tried to get a sense of the size of the reservoir by systematically examining entire organs during autopsies.

Lung cancer

Pathologists routinely stumble on lung cancers while performing autopsies on patients who have died for other reasons. The notion that such "surprise" cases suggest a reservoir of undetected lung cancer was first raised by Yale researchers almost 20 years ago.[18] They examined the autopsy reports of patients, generally over age 60, who died at Yale–New Haven Hospital and who were not known to have had lung cancer during life. The rate of surprise cases of lung cancer in these autopsies was 10 times the rate of lung cancer diagnosed in the general population of Connecticut, as reported in the State Tumor Registry. The difference? In the autopsies, the pathologists were cutting the lung into sections and looking hard for cancer. In the registry, doctors were reporting cancer that had generally come to their attention because the patient had symptoms (e.g., cough, weight loss, hoarseness).

What does this mean? If pathologists found very few lung cancers in patients not known to have cancer in life, clinicians could expect that most small lung cancers they do find will progress to be the type of lung cancer we all fear. In fact, however, pathologists find a high incidence of lung cancers in patients not known to have cancer in life; therefore, clinicians need to recognize that many small lung cancers detected by CAT scan may be pseudodisease.

More scrutiny, more cancer

How much the pathologist finds is dependent to some extent on how hard he looks. To understand why, you need to understand how pathologists examine tissue. They remove the organ from the body and then cut it into very thin slices—about 5 microns (less than 1/500 of an inch) thick—to be examined under the microscope. Although pathologists look pretty carefully at every slice they examine, they cannot examine every possible slice. So they select a sample of slices to examine. As this drawing makes clear, it is always possible to select a slice that misses the cancer:

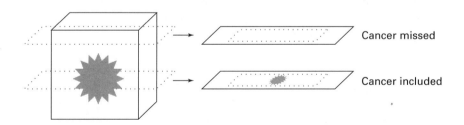

Imagine a pathologist trying to figure out how common surprise cancers are in patients not known to have cancer. He has no idea where to look.[19] The discovery of a cancer will then depend on its size and how many slices he looks at. Let's say the pathologist was looking for cancer in a small organ about the size of a sugar cube, 1 centimeter on a side. This cube could be cut into 2,000 slices, each of which is 5 microns thick. Typically, however, a pathologist examines 5, 10, maybe 20 slices. How many slices are enough? The answer affects both how often cancers are found and what size they are.

Thyroid cancer

The study that brought this relationship to my attention was done by pathologists in Finland who examined the thyroid gland in 101 autopsies.[20] Clinically, the thyroid—a gland in the lower neck that makes thyroid hormone, which in turn regulates a number of metabolic processes—is a rare site for cancer, in Finland as well as in the United States. But these investigators had learned that when other pathologists had carefully examined the thyroid, more cancer was found than expected.

So the investigators decided to look as hard as they could. They took sections of the thyroid about every 2 millimeters (less than 1/10 of an inch apart) and lo and behold, they found an amazing amount of cancer: over a third of the autopsied patients had thyroid cancer! However, many of the cancers were small, some as small as 0.2 mm in diameter—far smaller than the distance between the slices. They knew, therefore, that they must be missing many small cancers, and they had a pretty good idea just how many.

Their reasoning went something like this: because the slices were being made every 2 millimeters—no matter where they were made—any cancer larger than 2 mm in diameter could not be missed. You might visualize the situation like this:

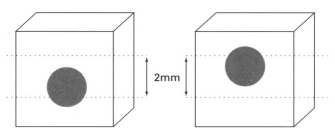

2 mm diameter cancer
will be included 100% of the time

But what about a 1 mm cancer? Sometimes they would catch it in the slice, sometimes it would be in between. If the slices were every 2 mm, roughly half the time they would expect to cut through a 1 mm cancer:

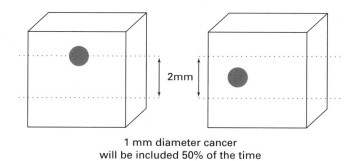

1 mm diameter cancer
will be included 50% of the time

The probability of detecting a small cancer is equal to its diameter divided by the distance between slices: in this case, 1 mm/2 mm, or 0.5. Therefore, they were only finding half of the 1 mm cancers. They were finding much smaller cancers as well, some as small as 0.2 mm. How many of these were they missing? Using the same reasoning, we calculate that they were finding 10 percent (0.2 mm/2 mm = 0.1)—which means they were missing 90 percent:

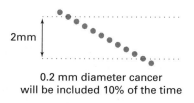

0.2 mm diameter cancer
will be included 10% of the time

Given the number of small cancers they did find and the number that they reasoned they missed, the researchers concluded that virtually everybody would have some evidence of thyroid cancer if examined carefully enough. So there is a bottomless reservoir of thyroid cancer. Put another way, we might say that the smallest forms of thyroid cancer are so common that they should be regarded as normal.

Although the thyroid is not aggressively biopsied in patients who display no signs or symptoms of cancer, this study highlights the kind of confusion that might occur were it to be. More important, the study provides a sense of how fuzzy the cancer versus normal tissue distinction can be when one is trying to diagnose cancer in small collections of cells. The problem is particularly acute in organs with a great deal of cellular activity: glands like the thyroid, prostate, and breast.

BREAST CANCERS YOU MIGHT RATHER NOT KNOW ABOUT

There is no blood test for breast cancer, but we do have mammography, an X-ray exam of the breast. The first mammograms, undertaken some 40 years ago, were relatively crude and were only able to detect relatively large cancers. Now mammography can detect tiny calcium-containing abnormalities mere millimeters across—about as big as this dot: • When biopsied, these so-called microcalcifications are often diagnosed as ductal carcinoma in situ (DCIS), a tiny form of breast cancer.

Look harder, find more DCIS

Figure 6 shows how looking harder has affected the frequency with which this form of breast cancer is found in women. As mammograms have become increasingly sensitive (and increasingly used), more and more DCIS has been found—ten times as much today as in 1973.[21]

As you may know, there is a lot of debate about what DCIS really means for women. There are debates about whether we are finding too much of it and debates about whether it should even be called cancer. But on one thing there is no debate: DCIS is being uniformly treated as if it were invasive cancer. Figure 7 compares current DCIS treatment with that for Stage 1 invasive breast cancer. Women with DCIS are a little less likely to receive radiation, but otherwise there is not much difference in treatment.

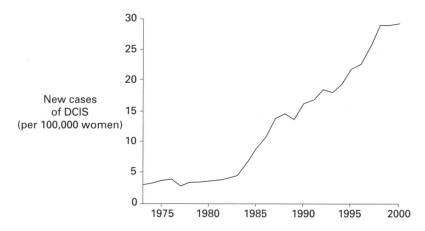

Figure 6. New cases of DCIS in the United States, 1973–2000.

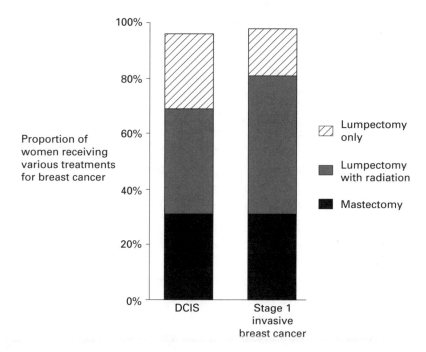

Figure 7. Treatments given women with DCIS and Stage 1 invasive breast cancer in the United States, 2000.

But is such aggressive treatment appropriate? Current clinical practice certainly conveys our belief that DCIS is destined to become invasive cancer. But is that really true?

Is DCIS really cancer?

If DCIS routinely progressed to invasive cancer, one would expect that finding it and treating it would lead to a decrease in the number of new cases of invasive breast cancer. Figure 8 shows the desired effect of finding and treating early cancer on the cancer statistics for a population. Start with the simplest case (Figure 8, top), where total cancer incidence—the rate of new cancer development—is stable over time. If finding more early-stage cancer helps, then the incidence of late-stage cancers should fall. Note that this phenomenon will be observed only if all the early cancers are destined to progress. Even if total cancer incidence is rising (Figure 8, bottom), one would still expect to see a substantial change in the incidence of late-stage cancers as more early-stage cancers are found and treated.

What is really happening in breast cancer incidence, however, is shown in Figure 9. We are finding more and more early-stage cancer, and yet there is no apparent effect on the rate of new cases of late-stage cancer. For context, the two dotted lines show the incidence of invasive cancer we might expect were all DCIS destined to progress (one assuming stable total incidence, the other assuming it rises 1 percent per year—as observed prior to the widespread use of mammography).[22] Because finding new cases of DCIS doesn't seem to change the incidence of invasive breast cancer, we must conclude either that early treatment doesn't help at all or—and much more likely—that many cases of DCIS are not destined to progress to invasive cancer.

This pattern of cancer incidence provides another line of evidence suggesting that most of what is diagnosed as DCIS is, in fact, pseudodisease. As we saw in Chapter 3, most women whose DCIS was missed at biopsy did not go on to develop invasive breast cancer; moreover, a DCIS diagnosis seems to have little, if any, impact on a woman's life expectancy. Now we have a third fact arguing that DCIS be considered pseudodis-

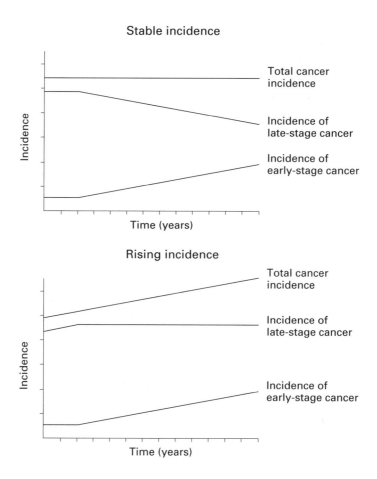

Figure 8.   Expected effect of finding more early-stage cancer on the incidence of late-stage cancer.

ease: despite a massive increase in the detection of this early cancer over the past 20 years, it is hard to see any effect on the number of cases of invasive breast cancer.

Almost half a million women have been diagnosed and treated for DCIS since the early 1980s—a diagnosis virtually unknown before then. This increase is the direct result of looking harder—in this case with "better"

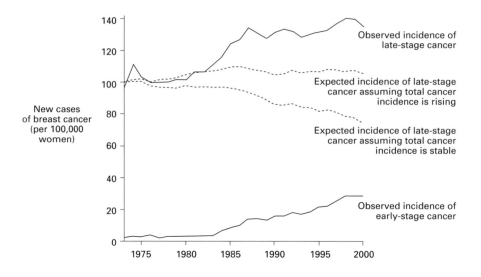

Figure 9.   Observed effect of finding more DCIS on the incidence of invasive breast cancer in the United States, 1973–2000.

mammography equipment. But I think you can see why it is a diagnosis that some women might reasonably prefer not to know about.

HOW MUCH MORE BREAST CANCER IS THERE TO FIND?

The existence of a considerable reservoir of prostate cancer is common knowledge among doctors. That the same might be true for breast cancer is less widely understood. Breast cancer feels like a scarier disease. In real terms, certainly, the stakes are higher. While prostate cancer is largely a disease of older men, breast cancer commonly involves middle-aged women. But as you can see, we may well be diagnosing cancer unnecessarily in the breast as well. And the problem could get a lot worse.

A few years ago a colleague and I published a structured review of a number of careful autopsy studies of the breast in women not known to have had breast cancer.[23] Table 4 summarizes the degree to which cancer—

Table 4   Autopsy series of women not known to have had breast cancer during life

Location	Women with breast cancer (all ages)	Middle-aged women with breast cancer[1]
Virginia (1973)	5.7%	—
California (1975)	4.5%	10%
Denmark (1984)	15.6%	—
California (1985)	8.9%	13%
Australia (1985)	13.5%	—
New Mexico (1987)	1.8%	7%
Denmark (1987)	15.6%	39%

SOURCE: H. G. Welch and W. C. Black, "Using Autopsy Series to Estimate the Disease 'Reservoir' for Ductal Carcinoma In Situ of the Breast: How Much More Breast Cancer Can We Find?" *Annals of Internal Medicine* 127 (1997): 1023–1028.

[1]The Virginia, Denmark 1984, and Australia studies did not differentiate by age. The middle-aged women in the California 1975 study were 50–70 years old; in the California 1985 study, 40–70; in the New Mexico study, 45–54; and in the Denmark 1987 study, 40–49.

both invasive breast cancer and DCIS—was found in each study, for both the total population and (where available) for those women we typically screen: middle-aged women. Two things about this table are striking. First, the reservoir of undetected breast cancer is substantial: a high proportion of these women have some evidence of breast cancer—mostly DCIS, the tiny form of breast cancer. In comparison, the lifetime risk of dying of breast cancer is less than 4 percent. Clearly, the potential to find more breast cancers than will ultimately matter to women is great.[24]

Also striking is the wide variation in results for the different studies. A number of reasons can be given. Although it is possible that the women studied had a different genetic risk for breast cancer, I doubt this explains much of the difference because almost all were of European descent. The differences in how much breast cancer was found could, however, be a function of how hard the pathologists looked—or in this case, how much of the breast they examined. The breast is a pretty big organ. Since they can't examine all of it under the microscope, pathologists must decide how much to look at. The New Mexico study, for example, looked at 9 microscope slides per breast, while the two Danish studies looked at an average of 95 and 275 slides per breast, respectively. Consequently, it is not surprising that the Danes found more breast cancer.

Then too, the numbers might be different simply because the pathologists were different. Different pathologists have different standards for diagnosing cancer—a topic sufficiently important that I devote the next chapter to it.

SUMMARY

I remember when I first learned that if people were examined carefully enough at death, virtually everybody would show some evidence of thyroid cancer. At the time my daughter, who was in elementary school, was trying to make sense of the riddle "If a tree falls in the woods and no one hears it, does it make a sound?" Somehow that riddle had passed me by during my own childhood, but learning it made me think about the analogous riddle of early cancer detection: "If someone is found to have abnormal cells at death and no one knew about it during their life, did the person have cancer?"

In the last two chapters I have explored some of the ambiguity in the word *cancer*. The answers to even the most basic questions, "How much cancer is there?" and "Who has it?," depend on the scrutiny of the observer. Because there is a substantial reservoir of undetected cancer, just being examined affects your chances of being told you have cancer. And the more carefully and systematically you are examined, the more likely it is that the cancers found will be cancers you would rather not know about.

Let me review the major points of this chapter. First, whenever doctors look harder, they find more cancer. Second, most of the "extra" cancers found are relatively small. Third, because they are small we can infer that many other small cancers are being missed. The reservoir of cancer is, therefore, potentially bottomless. So there you have it: all of us, at some point in our life, could probably be said to have cancer.

You know this is crazy. Only so many people die from cancer, and only

so many are ever bothered by symptoms. Could it be that our enthusiasm for cancer testing leads us to detect cancer in thousands of people
who would otherwise never be affected by the disease? And given the
uncertainty and fear associated with a cancer diagnosis and the harms
of treatment, isn't it possible that many would be better off simply not
knowing?

FIVE

Your pathologist may say it's cancer,
while others say it's not

The possibility that different pathologists could look at the same thing and make different diagnoses was not something I considered during my training. As medical residents, we always looked to the pathologist for the final answer on what was wrong with a patient. When faced with a diagnostic dilemma, we would even joke that "tissue was the issue" (that is, getting a specimen to send to pathology). Then, early in my academic career, I was invited to do a talk show on the local public radio station. One of the callers had been diagnosed with prostate cancer following a blood test for PSA (prostate specific antigen). The diagnosis was based on a biopsy that had been interpreted by a pathologist in Burlington, Vermont. The caller had asked another pathologist in Boston for a second opinion. She reviewed the specimens and concluded he did not have prostate cancer. The caller wanted to know what he should do. I had no idea what to say.

Let me say at the outset that pathologists have a difficult job. They are the doctors who examine tissue specimens under a microscope and decide whether what they see is cancer. They may even specialize and become experts on certain types of cancer. The rest of us, doctors and patients alike, traditionally see pathologists as the "gold standard" in cancer diagnosis: they have the final say on the question of who has and who does not have cancer.

My fear is that by the end of this chapter you will conclude that pathologists are not up to this job. That is certainly not my intent. Rather, my aim is simply to delineate the problem they face: while some specimens are clearly cancer and some are clearly normal, many specimens fall somewhere in between. It is on these specimens that pathologists are bound to disagree. I also want to pose a couple of questions for the rest of us: Are we expecting too much of pathologists? Is it reasonable to expect them *always* to be right?

MAKING A DIAGNOSIS

The challenge pathologists face became obvious to me a few years ago. An elderly man had come to our emergency room because he was getting very short of breath. He had very little oxygen in his blood, considerable swelling in his legs, and the sound of fluid in his lungs. Most commonly, these symptoms would be the result of heart failure. To confirm the diagnosis, I ordered a chest X-ray. That confirmed fluid in the lungs and demonstrated that the heart was enlarged (and therefore failing), but it also showed a large mass in the upper part of the right lung.

This is often the way we discover lung cancer: we take a chest X-ray for some other reason and find a mass. The X-ray, combined with the fact that this man was a smoker, made the diagnosis of lung cancer particularly likely. A CAT scan showed abnormalities in the liver and in the lymph nodes next to the lungs. These potential metastases gave further support to the diagnosis of lung cancer. Although the need for further tests might be questionable, our pulmonologist (a lung specialist) wanted to be sure. She decided to get a biopsy. This procedure involved passing a flexible fiber-optic scope through the patient's trachea (windpipe) into one of its branches, inserting a needle through the wall of the trachea into the lung, and withdrawing a tiny piece of the mass for the pathologist to examine.

Because I was this patient's primary care doctor, I went to watch. Others present included the pulmonologist, a pulmonologist-in-training, a nurse, and one of our pathologists, who would look at tissue samples while the scope was still in the patient's lungs. If he saw cancer, the procedure would be over. If he didn't, the pulmonologist would insert the needle in a slightly different direction and take another sample. Because everybody was anxious to get the biopsy over with—both because of the fragile condition of the patient and because they had other work to do—there was some pressure on the pathologist. After the patient was attached to various monitors and sedated, the procedure began.

The pulmonologist introduced the scope into the patient's trachea without any difficulty. Guided by the CAT scan, she directed it to the upper part of the right lung. (The scope had a camera, so we could all watch on a video monitor.) She inserted the needle and withdrew some tissue for the pathologist to examine. While the rest of us waited, the pathologist put the tissue on a glass slide and looked at it through the microscope. He saw no cancer. The pulmonologist took another sample. We waited again. This time he saw abnormal cells, but they might just be inflammation. On the monitor overhead, we saw some bleeding at the biopsy site. The patient began to cough. Another biopsy was taken. The pathologist studied the third slide. There was more bleeding, and more coughing. The pulmonologist looked impatient, even a little nervous. She wanted to wrap up this procedure. Then the long-awaited announcement: "Yeah, there's cancer here."

We were done. The scope was removed, the group disbanded, and the patient went to the recovery room. I was curious about the apparent uncertainty and went with the pathologist to his office to examine the tissue under more leisurely conditions. Here he had a microscope with which we could both examine the same area at the same time. He could show me the full range of cells—those that were normal, those that were inflamed, and those that were cancer—and I could ask questions. The normal was easy; but I was having trouble with the distinction between inflammation and cancer. So was the pathologist—and he was honest about it. He now, on second viewing, decided that his original diagnosis was premature. He asked another pathologist to review the slides. And they agreed: given only the cells they had in front of them, all they could say was that it might be lung cancer, but it might not.

THE PATHOLOGIST'S JOB

This story highlights three aspects of decision making in pathology. First, the pathologist has potentially a lot of material to look at. How much is actually examined—that is, how many cells are collected and how many are then evaluated—can affect whether cancer is diagnosed. As we saw in the previous chapter, this issue is particularly relevant to how many small cancers are detected.

Second, a pathologist's decision is frequently made under pressure. Time is often an issue: the doctors taking the biopsy are often waiting for the pathologist's decision so they can plan their next step. Even if there isn't a time constraint, the pathologist always has other specimens to look at. There is also the pressure of being right. Although no pathologist wants to make the diagnosis of cancer unnecessarily, pathologists are much more concerned about "missing" a cancer diagnosis. Most, if not all, pathologists have at least one story of a missed cancer—a patient whose biopsy was "normal" but who went on to die of cancer. On the other hand, it is impossible to know how often cancer is unnecessarily diagnosed, since anything called cancer is typically treated. In these cases, rather than saying that a cancer diagnosis was inaccurate or unnecessary, we come to a very different conclusion: the treatment was successful. Consequently, there is a strong incentive to overdiagnose. When in doubt, it is safest to call an abnormality cancer.

Finally, the diagnosis of cancer is inherently subjective: it involves a human judgment. As was mentioned in the introduction, the pathologist's decisions are based on both the appearance of individual cells and the organization of the cells (called the microscopic architecture). The less individual cells look like the normal cells found in the organ, the more likely it is cancer. The more individual cells vary in size and shape, the more likely it is cancer. And the more the pathologist sees individual cells in the midst of dividing, the more likely it is cancer. The microscopic architecture is important because it provides information about how invasive the cells are as a unit and how successfully the body is reacting to them (the host response). Growths that appear to be walled off from surrounding tissue—as if in a cocoon—are less likely to be cancer. Growths that appear to extend into surrounding tissue and invade nearby blood vessels are more likely to be cancer.

The operative word here is *appear:* the pathologic diagnosis of cancer depends on an individual's judgment about a visual image. It is therefore not surprising that one pathologist might see one thing, while another might see something else. This is not to say that all pathologists will see something different—and make completely different diagnoses—only that the potential for disagreement exists.

To consider the problem of disagreement, look at this pair of circles:

Would everyone you know agree on which one is black? Unless you have very odd acquaintances, disagreement is extremely unlikely here.

Now take a look at another two circles:

If you had to choose one "gray" one, which would it be? Here, disagreement seems quite likely.

Now let's say that anything "dark gray or darker" is a cancer. With this knowledge, consider these five "cases":

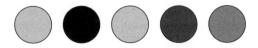

Would everyone you know agree on how many of these cases are cancer? I doubt it. Some might decide there is one case of cancer, some might say two cases, and some might even say five.

Normal		Invasive Cancer
Normal breast	Atypical ductal hyperplasia → Ductal carcinoma in-situ	Breast cancer
Normal cervix	ASCUS[1] → Squamous intraepithelial lesion → Carcinoma in situ	Cervical cancer
Normal colon	Hyperplastic polyp → Tubular adenoma → Villous adenoma	Colon cancer
Normal lung	Atypical adenomatous hyperplasia → Bronchioloalveolar carcinoma	Lung cancer
Normal skin	Atypical nevus → Melanocytic nevus → Dysplastic nevus	Melanoma
Normal prostate	Prostatic hyperplasia → Prostatic intraepithelial neoplasia	Prostate cancer

[1]ASCUS = atypical squamous cells of unknown significance.

Figure 10.   The spectrum from normal to cancer.

In a simple black and white world, a diagnosis would involve only two assessments: normal and cancer. There would be no room for disagreement. In the real world, however, there is a spectrum of abnormalities— a huge gray area—between normal cells and invasive cancer. Pathologists have long recognized that this gray area exists. They have created a range of diagnoses to fill the gap between normal and cancer for almost every organ in the body. Some of the names given the shades of gray for selected organs appear in Figure 10. Don't pay too much attention to the names themselves, because different pathologists use different nomenclature in the gray zone. My main interest is that you too recognize that these in-between abnormalities exist.

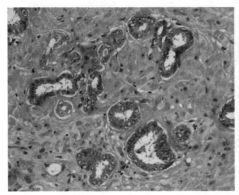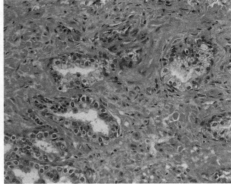

Figure 11.   Microscopic views of the prostate gland (*left*, cancer; *right*, noncancer).

Naturally, the existence of a gray zone makes disagreement more likely. While the distinction between invasive cancer and normal tissue is relatively straightforward, it is more difficult to distinguish among the abnormalities in between. Therefore, although pathologists are likely to agree about what is an obvious cancer and what is obviously normal, they may not agree on whether or not subtle cellular abnormalities constitute early cancer. And those are exactly the kinds of abnormalities that are found when we go looking for cancer in healthy people.

The pathologic diagnosis of cancer depends, essentially, on a subjective judgment, as the classic pathology textbook that many of us used in medical school makes clear: "Despite man's ingenuity in inventing amazingly sophisticated instrumentation, the anatomic diagnosis of neoplasms is largely accomplished by 'eyeballing.' In some part a science, and in large part an art, it is heavily dependent on the brain behind the eyes behind the microscope."[1] It is therefore not surprising that one pathologist might see one thing while another sees something else.

To get a feel for the problem, take a look at Figure 11, which shows two microscopic views of the prostate: the left frame is cancer, the right is not.[2] Of course, pathologists undergo lengthy training to know what to look for. They would know to focus on the round structures (the microscopic glands in the prostate) and ignore the lacy red background (the intervening connective tissue). They would see that the architecture—the size, shape, and configuration of these glands—was not that different in the two frames. But they would notice that the cells lining the glands were a darker blue on the left than on the right. They would also notice that the cells on the left have more material in their center—the nucleus, where the cell's reproductive machinery is housed. These are signs of cancer. But how dark do cells need to be before a pathologist calls them cancer? And how much extra material does there need to be? As these pictures make clear, the visual interpretation required to make the diagnosis of cancer can be very delicate indeed.

OBSERVER VARIATION: WHAT IS THE DIAGNOSIS?

The idea that doctors do not always agree about correct treatment is well known. Some patients, in fact, shop doctors until they find one who recommends the therapy they want. But the idea that pathologists may disagree about a diagnosis is less familiar. To their credit, the pathology community has been studying this issue.

Two basic problems could lead pathologists to disagree about a diagnosis: either they look at different things or they look at the same thing and see something different. Recall that biopsy specimens (generally obtained by a surgeon or radiologist) are sent to the pathologist, who then takes several thin slices of tissue and places them on glass slides to examine under the microscope. If pathologists examine different slices, they may arrive at different diagnoses. And, as suggested in Chapter 4, if they look at more slices, they may be more likely to diagnose cancer. The studies of how well pathologists agree, however, do not investigate this source of disagreement. Instead, they take the slice as their starting point and make sure the pathologists are looking at the same thing. Thus they address the question "Do pathologists agree about what they see?"

Prostate cancer

Researchers at the Boston VA Hospital asked eight experienced pathologists (each with more than 10 years of experience) to examine 321 needle biopsies of the prostate.[3] The biopsies were consecutive; that is, once the research project started, a specimen from every man who had a prostate biopsy in the hospital was included. In other words, the specimens were not selected because they were unusual (e.g., especially challenging diagnoses); rather, they were representative of prostate biopsies in general.

All eight pathologists offered the same diagnosis for the majority of biopsies: most (239 cases) were not cancer, while 17 biopsies did turn up cancer.[4] But in 65 biopsies—20 percent of the cases—some of the pathologists made a cancer diagnosis, while others did not. In other words, there were a lot of split decisions.

Researchers at Johns Hopkins University took another approach to obtain biopsy specimens.[5] Instead of using consecutive cases, they attempted to represent the full diagnostic spectrum of prostate cancer by carefully selecting 25 specimens from their pathology collection.[6] They then recruited seven expert pathologists from major American teaching hospitals, including Hopkins itself, Stanford, the University of Texas, M. D. Anderson Cancer Center, Barnes Hospital in St. Louis, and the Armed Forces Institute of Pathology in Washington, D.C. Because the researchers wanted to make sure all the pathologists were looking at the same cells, they either circled the target area (where the abnormality was) or used tape to mask off the irrelevant portion of the slide.

For 13 of the 25 specimens the pathologists agreed that there was no cancer, and on one they agreed that cancer was present. For the remaining 11 specimens, however, the diagnosis was split: 6 yes to 1 no (3 specimens); 5 to 2 (1 specimen); 4 to 3 (1 specimen); 3 to 4 (2 specimens); 2 to 5 (1 specimen); and 1 to 6 (3 specimens). Remember: these pathologists were all selected because of their expertise. Yet almost half of the cases were split decisions, and in only one instance was a diagnosis of cancer unanimous.[7]

These two studies demonstrate a disturbing truth: whether or not you are *told* you have prostate cancer depends on who your pathologist is. Unfortunately, these studies don't tell us the source of disagreement. Do pathologists have different standards for diagnosing cancer, or do they all simply make mistakes?

Melanoma

Disagreement among pathologists has also been examined in melanoma, the most feared form of skin cancer. Unfortunately, even under the microscope, melanoma can be difficult to distinguish from a benign mole, known as a melanocytic nevus. To learn more about how pathologists make this distinction, the National Institutes of Health convened a group of eight pathologists, all experts in skin cancer.[8] Each was asked to contribute five skin biopsy specimens that he or she considered a classic case of either melanoma or a melanocytic nevus. Thirty-seven specimens were selected and stripped of all identification. Each pathologist was then asked to review all 37 specimens—including those personally submitted.

This study was exceptionally well done. The investigators reported the diagnosis given each specimen by each pathologist (37 × 8 = 296 diagnoses). Since that's a lot of information, I needed an easy way to show it. My solution was to use a grid depicting specimens in columns and pathologists in rows.

Figure 12 illustrates the 13 skin specimens for which all eight pathologists agreed that melanoma was either present or absent. A shaded square represents a cancer diagnosis, a clear square a diagnosis of no cancer. So the vertical strips indicate perfect agreement about the diagnosis: in this case, 5 were cancer, 8 were not.

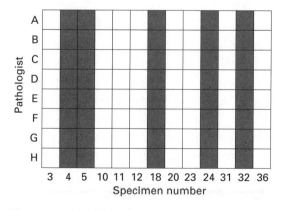

Figure 12.   Grid of 13 skin specimens in which pathologists *agreed* whether melanoma was present.

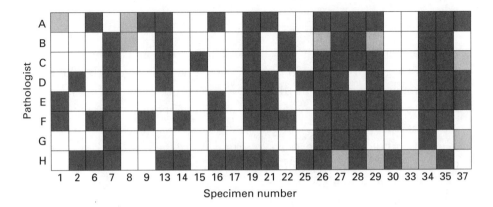

Figure 13. Grid of 24 skin specimens in which pathologists *disagreed* whether melanoma was present.

But that leaves 24 skin specimens. And here the grid looks more like a checker board (Figure 13). In some specimens almost all the pathologists agreed that cancer was present (specimen 7, for example), while in others almost all agreed that there was no cancer (specimen 15, for example). But in many cases the disagreement is more widespread, with some pathologists saying cancer, others saying no cancer, and some saying they're not sure (the lighter gray squares).

Figure 13 also provides some insight into *why* pathologists disagree. Look at that checkerboard again, but this time focus on the rows. Note that pathologist G made a melanoma diagnosis in only 5 specimens, while pathologist F did so in 16 specimens. Among these questionable specimens, pathologist F was more than three times as likely to diagnose melanoma as pathologist G. This suggests that the reason for disagreement is not simply that pathologists make random mistakes, but that different pathologists have different standards for calling an abnormality cancer. In other words, one reason pathologists disagree is that some have a greater tendency to diagnose cancer than others.

Because melanoma seems to be increasingly common, doctors are looking for it more aggressively and performing more skin biopsies (some would argue that melanoma is becoming more common *because* doctors are looking for it more aggressively; more on this in Chapter 8). Consequently, pathologists are looking at more and more skin biopsies trying to decide whether melanoma is present. And just like with prostate cancer, whether you are told you have melanoma will in part depend on who your pathologist is.

Breast cancer

Diagnostic disagreement has also been documented in breast cancer. In one study, six pathologists who specialize in breast pathology each examined the same set of 24 specimens.[9] These specimens were "close calls": none were normal, yet none were big, obvious cancers; instead they were all "proliferative lesions," meaning that all had areas where cells were rapidly reproducing (a not uncommon occurrence in a gland such as the breast).

In these small lesions the cancer (called ductal carcinoma in situ, or DCIS) versus noncancer (ductal hyperplasia or ductal atypia) distinction can be extremely subtle.[10] These pathologists were therefore taking on a considerable challenge—and they did their best to prepare for it. First they limited themselves to one of three diagnostic categories, which would render agreement more likely. Next they developed a written set of guidelines and diagrams on the criteria for these three diagnoses. They then sat down as a group and reviewed a set of five teaching slides in each diagnostic category. Finally they evaluated the set of 24 study slides, which were carefully taped to ensure that each pathologist would look at the same area of the slide.

Despite this effort, there was disagreement about whether or not DCIS was present in 8 of the 24 specimens. Figure 14 shows the grid for all 24 specimens. Shaded squares represent a DCIS diagnosis; clear squares represent a diagnosis of no cancer. Note that there was complete agreement that 14 specimens were not DCIS and that 2 specimens were DCIS (numbers 5 and 23). That leaves 8 specimens—fully one-third—in which the pathologists did not agree on the presence or absence of cancer. And once again there is evidence that the propensity to diagnose cancer varied among the pathologists. Pathologist C made a cancer diagnosis in 12.5 per-

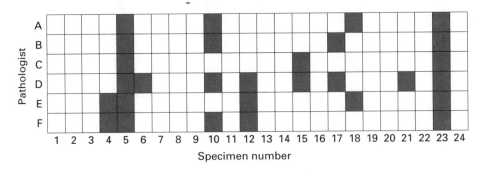

Figure 14.   Grid of 24 breast specimens in which pathologists considered whether DCIS was present.

cent of the specimens (3 in 24), while pathologist D found cancer in 33 percent of the specimens (8 in 24).

Two aspects of this study must be considered to put it in proper perspective. On one hand, these pathologists were studying only "close calls"—the toughest cases. One would expect better results in real life, where these in-between cells would be balanced out by big invasive breast cancers and normal breast tissue. On the other hand, in real life pathologists don't meet to establish criteria and look at training slides, nor is the specimen masked to make sure everyone is looking at the same cells. So in a real-world situation the disagreement about these cases would have been more pronounced.

Perhaps the best example of real life is a community-based study of pathologists that was conducted in New Hampshire.[11] Thirty slides were randomly selected from a statewide pathology database and sent out to 26 pathologists. In 16 of the 30 slides, at least one pathologist identified cancer. But in only 8 cases did all 26 pathologists agree that cancer was present[12]—and in half of those, there was disagreement about whether the cancer was invasive or not.

A little perspective

I don't want to end this discussion without reiterating that these studies do not necessarily represent typical practice; specifically, the results often overstate the problem of pathologist disagreement. The Hopkins prostate cancer study, for example, selected slides to "represent the full diagnostic spectrum," which means that odd (or difficult) diagnoses are likely overrepresented relative to real-life practice. Tougher cases could be overrepresented in the melanoma study as well, despite its express intent of examining "classic cases." And the first breast cancer study I described specifically chose specimens that were close calls.

Of all the studies discussed, only the VA prostate cancer and New Hampshire breast cancer studies are truly population-based, representing a spectrum of actual, real-world cases—a typical veteran undergoing prostate biopsy in Boston and a typical woman undergoing breast biopsy in New Hampshire. From these we get some sense of the size of the gray zone in real life, with disagreement in roughly a fifth of the prostate cases (65/321) and a quarter of the breast biopsies (8/30).[13]

EARLY DETECTION: SUBTLE ABNORMALITIES, NOT SO SUBTLE PROBLEMS

In the search for early cancers, the pathologist becomes an important variable in the diagnostic equation. Not only, as we have seen, is there an element of chance in whether a small abnormality is found to begin with; but once one is found, pathologists may not agree about what to call it. Consequently, in the case of small cancers at least, whether or not you are told you have cancer depends on who interprets the slide, as well as on how hard they look.

This was not always the case. In the past, pathologists were sent growths that were large enough to be felt by hand (that's how most cancers were found). The invasion of surrounding tissue was evident to the naked eye. Many patients already had metastases. The diagnosis was unambiguous. Now, pathologists are sent growths so small that they are evident only on special imaging tests. Or there's no growth at all, instead organs are biopsied at random because of an abnormality in a blood test (such as a PSA).

Consider a baseball-sized growth that the surgeon had difficulty removing because it was invading the surrounding normal tissue. Under the microscope, lots of bizarre cells can be seen; it is clear that collections of these cells are invading the surrounding healthy tissue. The imaging test shows abnormalities in other organs. I am confident you could ask 100 pathologists and get the same answer: it's cancer.

Now consider the other extreme. There is no growth at all, just an abnormal blood test. If there is cancer at all, it's like finding a needle in a haystack. A sample of tissue is taken. There are some big cells, but not many. Let's say the tissue is from a gland—an organ where cells normally divide frequently. There may be a small collection of cells in a duct, but there is no appearance of invasion. Is it cancer? I am confident you will get varying answers from pathologists. As we look for earlier (and thus more subtle) forms of cancer, the problem of diagnostic disagreement is bound to increase.

Perhaps the real problem lies in the task itself. We can't expect pathologists to look at every cell—nor would we want them to. And we can't expect them to accurately predict the outcome of a dynamic multistep process (a cancer bound to spread and cause problems) based on a single static observation (the appearance of a few cells under a microscope). As long as our approach remains as it is, the process of early cancer diagnosis is bound to be haphazard.

SUMMARY

Whether or not you are told you have cancer depends in part on who your pathologist is. And being told you have cancer can change your life. Men who are told they have prostate cancer are likely to have a radical prostatectomy or get radiation. Individuals who are told they have melanoma are likely to have wide excisions and frequent follow-up exams. And women who are told they have breast cancer are likely to have a mastectomy or get radiation. In short, the pathologist's decision triggers a whole set of actions. Do they know what they are doing?

I think they do, most of the time. Pathologists do agree about big, obvious cancers. They also agree on what is normal tissue. But there is a fair amount in between: small cellular abnormalities that pathologists are bound to disagree about. These abnormalities typically reach the pathologist only after you have been tested for early cancer. And the more cancer testing you undergo, the more likely it is you will have an abnormality that pathologists will disagree about.

If that talk show caller who received two different diagnoses from two different pathologists were to call me today, I know what I would say. It may sound odd, but I believe he is better off than a person who has a cancer the pathologists agree on. Disagreement is information: it tells you that the abnormality you have is subtle. That means that the chances are good that it's not a lethal cancer, that your prognosis is good. Maybe it is an abnormality that should simply be watched.

SIX

Your doctor may get distracted from other issues that are more important to you

Many people go through cancer testing and experience none of the problems discussed in the foregoing chapters. They have normal results: no ambiguity, no pseudodisease, no cancer at all. Other than the reassurance that they are cancer free, these people have gained nothing from the process. Nor, most would say, have they lost anything in the process.

But I'm beginning to wonder whether that is true. Scheduled health maintenance—routine questionnaires, examinations, and tests given to people without symptoms—is an increasingly prominent part of American medicine. Most of our maintenance work involves testing for diseases, such as cancer. We order tests, describe them to patients, and do whatever is needed to prepare patients for them. When the tests are completed, we have to find the results, interpret the results, and then communicate them to patients. All this takes time—which must come from somewhere. I fear that "somewhere" is the time doctors used to spend paying attention to issues their patients wanted to talk about.

I see this problem as involving not just cancer testing but routine testing in general. Still, it is one more downside that you should consider as you contemplate testing for cancer. I should add, moreover, that the only evidence I have for this problem comes from my own observations. I know of no research on the subject. So consider this chapter with particular skepticism: if it doesn't make sense or jibe with your own experience in some way, feel free to discount it. All I ask is that you give some thought to how doctors might best spend their time with you.

THE PREVENTION MODEL

The theory

Sometime, take a look at the owner's manual of your car. Toward the back you'll find a chart for scheduled maintenance—telling you how often to have your oil changed, how often to replace spark plugs and air filters, how often to adjust the valve clearance and the idle speed, and how often to inspect such things as exhaust pipes, brake lines, steering linkage, and the transaxle. In fact, the manual for my Toyota Tercel has two charts: one for normal driving conditions and one for severe.

Medicine is moving in this direction. We have charts recommending scheduled maintenance for human beings, with different charts for different models: the scheduled maintenance for men, for example, is different from that for women. The recommended maintenance changes with age. Children have their own set of charts.[1] There are even charts for patients with specific diseases—diabetes, emphysema, and heart disease. Here, for example, is a set of recommendations for a healthy middle-aged male: "Provide nutritional and activity counseling every two years. Do a pain assessment every year. Check cholesterol every five years. Screen for alcohol use, depression, colon cancer every year. Ask about tobacco use every visit and provide counseling. Give flu vaccine annually, pneumococcal pneumonia vaccine at least once. Assess risk of Hepatitis C. Offer PSA (prostate specific antigen) testing, but counsel that we don't know if it helps people and we do know that some get hurt." The maintenance list for women is a little longer, the list for anyone with diabetes and heart disease considerably longer.

The practice

To give a sense of how routine maintenance works in practice, let me tell you about a typical clinic visit at the VA. Before I have even seen a patient, he has been weighed and has had his blood pressure and pulse taken. He has also responded to a number of brief questionnaires: about depression, hepatitis risk factors, pain, and alcohol use. When I'm ready to see him, I find him in the waiting area and walk with him back to my exam room. (Walking with a patient isn't simply a nice thing to do; it's one of the most important parts of the physical exam. It provides information about the patient's hips, knees, nervous system, and cardiovascular conditioning.)

Generally, I have already called up his medical record on the computer (I try to do this between patients). The electronic medical record is actually a complex set of interactive databases, but it opens up on a patient summary page. This page lists the patient's medical problems, medicines, recent appointments, and a list of "clinical reminders"—largely preventive interventions such as vaccinations and screening tests. Next to an intervention will be either the date it was last performed or the words DUE NOW (which most of my colleagues and I read as DO NOW).

So even without talking to the patient, I have a fair amount of information in front of me. (Actually, we have had a chance to talk during the walk to the exam room—in the summer generally about the Red Sox, in the winter generally about driving conditions. This chatting is important, both to reestablish the relationship and to learn about a patient's state of mind.) There is the list of things to do, as well as several paper questionnaires to review. For most patients there is also other information to consider: the results of tests ordered during a previous visit or things I made a note of that I wanted to check at the next visit. In short, I have an agenda—items I want to check off.

Of course, the patient (and/or his wife) often has things he wants to talk about—questions about problems he is experiencing, questions about his medications, or questions about health stories he has heard in the news. Often the list of things he wants to talk about is conceptual, but sometimes it's written out. Either way, the patient has an agenda as well.

Not surprisingly, our two agendas may compete with each other. Although I try to be sensitive to the forces at work, I know I'm not always successful. I try not to start with *my* list, but it does weigh on me. Some patients seem to be sensitive to the tension as well—not wanting to start *their* list until I'm through with mine, believing that my list is somehow more important. Others are not so sensitive. With them I find I may interrupt the conversation to check some items off my list.

Effect of more testing

The more testing there is, the more ends up on my list. Tests need to be ordered, some of which require that other tests be done first.[2] Some require instruction, such as the fecal occult blood test done at home. Once tests are completed, I go over the results with the patient. Even if the test is normal, some people need considerable reassurance that the test didn't miss something or that there isn't some "better test" out there somewhere. Then there is the question of when the test should be done again, a question that generally has no satisfactory answer.

And the minute there is an abnormal test, there's more to do. If a patient has a positive fecal occult blood test, for example, I usually order a colonoscopy. This test uses a long, flexible fiber-optic tube, which is introduced into the rectum and then advanced through the length of the large intestine (some three to five feet). To prepare patients for this test, I describe both the test and what they will need to do to prepare for it: drink a large volume of special solution that will clean out their colon, requiring that they be near a toilet for a few hours. Roughly half the time the colonoscopy will detect some abnormality—most commonly, a few benign growths called polyps or adenomas. If so, the question arises of when—or whether—another colonoscopy should be performed in the future.[3] I like to review the recommendation of the gastroenterologist (the doctor performing the test) and note it in the record. If a future colonoscopy is recommended, it must be decided whether to continue with fecal occult blood testing in the interim. It's easy to forget that this patient's primary problem may be trouble breathing or back pain, something unrelated to the testing.

OUT OF BALANCE

Of course, the VA is not typical of American medicine. For one thing, the electronic medical record at the VA and in other comprehensive health systems, such as Kaiser-Permanente, is more advanced and complete than that used in a typical private practice. It allows doctors to establish reminder systems prompting them to do various things in various circumstances. Furthermore, health maintenance interventions have traditionally been highly valued in these comprehensive health systems—a fact reflected in the very term HMO, "health maintenance organization." Although this tradition may be weaker in the private sector (and the process more haphazard), the forces promoting scheduled health maintenance have influenced all of American medicine.

The problem is that promotion of scheduled health maintenance expands the physician agenda. The effect is both direct—additional time is required whenever another test is added—and indirect, by which I mean all the downstream consequences: abnormalities identified by testing will require further evaluation and attention. Add the fact that many patients have prior medical problems that also require routine tasks, and it's easy to see how the typical 15- to 20-minute clinic visit can become dominated by the physician agenda, leaving little time for the patient's concerns.[4]

Of course, the problem of competing agendas has always been with us. What is changing is the size of the physician agenda. And what has not changed is the length of a typical clinic visit, which has remained between 15 and 20 minutes for the past 10 years.[5] The patient agenda had to give, resulting in a physician-patient encounter that is out of balance.

There are those who see medicine as a purely objective science, in which patients' subjective experience and concerns are unimportant. Although these people may believe that doctors can learn everything they need to know from diagnostic tests, this is not the case. In fact, we identify most important medical problems by listening to our patients, not from special tests. Patients often have a story to tell, and listening to it takes time. They may not start with their most important complaint. They may be afraid to share what they find most worrisome. They may test the water to see how the doctor responds, taking their time to get to what is really bothering them. If doctors take the time to listen carefully to these concerns and sort through them, they may arrive at new diagnoses or be more confident that patients are in fact well. And if doctors take the time to react to these concerns and explain their thinking, they may be better able to reassure patients. Both are important—both the listening and the talking.

But patients often have other things on their agenda. They may have questions about their medications or about side effects they are experiencing. They may want advice about chronic conditions such as back pain, digestive problems, or sexual dysfunction. They may need to share something about their social situation—their employment, their marriage, their family dynamics—areas in which change, conflict, and loss can adversely affect not only mental health but physical health as well. Taking the time to answer questions, suggest strategies for coping with chronic conditions, and bear witness to human suffering is an important part of the therapeutic role of a physician.

SUMMARY

In the past, doctors saw patients without having a preset agenda. Now, we increasingly have one: "You are due for A, B, and C, and we also recommend that everyone does X." And much of that agenda relates to screening. From the physician's perspective, scheduled maintenance has some appeal. It is a concrete service that identifies problems that can be acted on. Discussing patient concerns, in contrast, can feel ethereal and frequently concludes with sympathy, not a definite plan. If patients do not express strong preferences for the latter, doctors often gravitate to the former.

In this brief chapter I have introduced the problem as I see it. Routine testing is really a concern for what could happen in the future. And worrying about what might matter in the future can distract your doctor from what matters now. The more time we spend ordering tests and following up on abnormal results, the less time we spend dealing with things that concern you now.

Of course, a balance can be found. I'm not suggesting we abandon all scheduled health maintenance and restrict ourselves to addressing current patient concerns. We can certainly do some of both. But I do want you to consider that even if there were no other downsides to cancer testing—that is, if it could only be beneficial—it still might distract from other, more useful activities. I also want you to be aware that testing in general increasingly dominates the physician-patient encounter. In the next chapter, I'll tell you why.

PART II

BECOMING A BETTER-EDUCATED CONSUMER

SEVEN *Understand the culture of medicine (and why we are pushed to test)*

In the foregoing chapters I have described some of the basic principles of testing asymptomatic people for cancer and tried to explain the downsides of the process. These data demonstrate that cancer testing is a double-edged sword. Rather than being a "no-brainer," the decision about whether to get tested involves a genuine choice.

Knowledge is the key to making good decisions. And there is more to knowledge than simply knowing today's facts. Part of being knowledge-able involves the ability to interpret new information in the future. It is also important to understand what we will likely never know. And because cancer testing has benefits and harms that different people feel differently about, an especially critical part of being knowledgeable involves knowing yourself. In the remaining chapters, I want to help you develop these skills.

The first step in developing the knowledge needed to make decisions about medical treatment is to understand the culture you are working with—in this case, the culture of medicine. You have to have a feel for the forces that influence doctors and a sense of how doctors see the world. It is also worth knowing something about other important players—specifically, health care managers and researchers. Better understanding the medical culture will not only give insight into why doctors do what they do, but it will also explain why people should develop a healthy skepticism and ask questions about the information they are given.

YOUR DOCTOR'S NIGHTMARE

A few years ago, a close friend of mine was taken to court for failure to diagnose prostate cancer. Joel was sued by a middle-aged man who had seen him on two occasions. Both times the patient had come for a routine checkup. Joel asked him if he had any complaints. He said he was fine. Joel checked his blood pressure; he listened to his lungs. Both were normal. He did a rectal exam, where the examiner inserts a finger into the rectum to feel both the prostate and the wall of the rectum, another potential cancer site. As is the case with many middle-aged men, the prostate was enlarged, but otherwise it was normal. On the first visit he also referred the man for a sigmoidoscopy, one of the screening tests for colorectal cancer. It too was normal.

Six months later the patient started having trouble urinating. He went to a urologist, a doctor who specializes in the male urinary system. The urologist repeated the rectal exam and felt the prostate. Now there was a growth. The urologist did a PSA test; it was sky high, suggesting a cancer that had spread beyond the prostate. He learned about the patient's previous visit with Joel and said, "If your doctor had done a PSA test six months ago, he would have saved your life."

At the risk of sounding like a stereotypic doctor defending the interests of his friend and profession, I will simply say that this is an egregious statement. First and foremost, the PSA test has never been demonstrated to save anyone's life. No one should suggest someone's life "would have been saved" without some evidence that the strategy works.

But even if PSA testing had been shown to work, the statement is still egregious, because it is far too definitive. If PSA testing worked, then yes, it is *possible* that the cancer might have been detected six months earlier, while it was treatable. Possible, but not certain—for other possibilities exist. First, the cancer may not even have been present six months earlier, in which case, of course, it could not have been detected by any test. Second, even if the cancer were present at the earlier visit, it is quite possible that it was not treatable.

Clearly, this patient had developed a very aggressive cancer. That's a terrible thing. Joel felt bad for him. So would I, and I'm sure you would too. Something very unfortunate had happened to another human being. But the urologist compounded the tragedy by doing another terrible thing: he played right into an increasingly destructive (and common) mind-set in our society, which is to assign blame. Something bad has happened, so someone must be at fault.

The case went to trial in a small town in Vermont. Experts on prostate cancer screening from the University of Connecticut and Harvard University testified about what we do and do not know about early detection, telling much the same story I related in Chapter 3. But then there was the local urologist telling the jury an emotional story: this particular doctor failed to diagnose a cancer. Add to that a real patient with advanced cancer, looking all the worse because he was suffering from the side effects of treatment. There were even courtroom theatrics. At one point, the patient's wife stood up, pointed at Joel, and yelled "murderer." I presume she was coached to do so, much as Joel was coached to bring his wife and daughter to court to help humanize him.

You can probably guess the rest of the story. The jury found for the plaintiff. Joel's lawyers felt that although a more rational verdict could almost certainly be obtained on appeal, the cost of the process would likely exceed the proposed award, and so the case was settled. Not surprisingly, Joel now orders more PSA tests. He refers more patients to urologists, they find more prostate cancer, and more patients suffer the side effects of therapy. The experience affected how Joel practices medicine. Not wanting to appear in a courtroom again, not wanting to be accused of failing to order a test, he orders more tests in general now. It makes sense. I don't know of any doctor who has had to appear in court because he *did* order a test.

FORCES THAT ENCOURAGE DOCTORS TO TEST

Because doctors are human, we don't always do exactly what we think is in the very best interest of the patient. Other forces influence our behavior. This is true for testing in general and cancer testing in particular. Recognizing these forces will help you respond to them.

Fear

The most obvious outside force in the practice of medicine is fear. Doctors are always worried about missing something and having someone else find it. This fear starts in medical school, where the physical exam becomes a sort of competition. Students are separated into two groups: those who hear extra heart sounds, detect small differences in reflexes, discern slight changes in the coloring of the tongue, and so forth—and those who don't. Being aware of such subtleties is equated with being a good doctor, missing them with being a substandard one. Almost all medical students want to be "good" doctors, and many worry that they aren't good enough. The response is predictable: look hard to find things wrong.

Of course, the fear of having another doctor tell you that you missed something pales in comparison to the fear of having a lawyer tell you you missed something. Whatever the reality of malpractice suits (and in fact, they are not as common or as serious as most think),[1] it is the perceived risk of being sued that drives doctors to practice defensive medicine. In particular, it drives us to do tests.

Doctors may be reluctant to acknowledge that we ever order tests for some reason other than the clinical needs of the patient. Consider what happens at my hospital's weekly medical conference, where the medical staff reviews the case of a specific patient.[2] One doctor tells the patient's story (most participants don't know anything about the patient in question), stopping at critical junctures to ask the other doctors' opinions. The basic questions are "What diagnoses would you consider given this information?" and "What would you do next?" The answer to the latter typically involves a diagnostic test.

It's a stimulating meeting. But there seems to be a discrepancy between what tests we *say* we would order and what tests we in fact *do* order in similar situations. Almost all doctors would agree that indiscriminate testing is not in a patient's best interest. And in an educational forum, with many trainees in attendance, senior staff tend to be quite parsimonious in the tests they suggest. Occasionally, however, someone will point out the charade: in the real world most of us order more tests. Why? The fear of malpractice.

Of all the things we can miss, nothing feels worse than missing a case of cancer. No matter how much a doctor knows about the problems of early cancer diagnosis—and many know a good deal—no one wants to hear the words "you missed a cancer." There is no counterbalancing force; no one ever hears the words "you diagnosed this cancer unnecessarily." And so we test.

Professional satisfaction

In general, we like to take actions that will help people. A century ago there was very little we could do to treat illness—the exception being surgery, which was sufficiently dangerous and painful to be reserved only for the most severe problems. The past hundred years have seen an explosion in the number of things we can do, particularly in terms of new medicines and tests. While most of these treatments have real value in selected situations, in many situations we turn to them largely because we can. CAT scans of the head, for example, which represented a tremendous advance in the management of severe head trauma, are now commonly used to evaluate headaches, where they have marginal value. Similarly, antidepressant medication, though a huge advance for the treatment of severe depression, is now dispensed in settings where its utility is far less obvious. We prescribe medicines and order tests both because tangible activity helps us feel productive and because it's expedient.

It is much easier to write a prescription or order a test than to talk about a difficult problem. Listening to patients can be hard. Their stories may be disorganized or tedious. They may repeat themselves, they may ramble. Worse yet, they may bring up problems that can't be solved. While medicine will continually advance, there will always be problems that have no solution. Frustrated by our inability to fix things, many doctors either ignore these problems, refer patients to other doctors (even when we are quite confident that they won't be able to solve the problem either), or order a test that is somehow connected—however tenuously—to the patient's complaint.

Routine testing is very comfortable. With it we are on the familiar ground of impressive technology, hard science, and apparently definitive findings. By ordering tests we feel like we are providing a concrete service, one with which few could find fault. At the same time, testing can be something that we hide behind: it conveys the illusion that something useful is being done. And by identifying actionable problems, it can provide a convenient distraction, allowing us to sidestep the more difficult problems that patients want to talk about.

In addition, we *like* to find disease: it's what we're trained to do. It isn't unusual to hear a doctor animatedly talking to a colleague about a recent diagnosis he or she has made. It's not bragging; it's the excitement of solving a puzzle. Diagnosing an early cancer is particularly satisfying because we are tempted to believe we are making an important difference in a person's life (something that may or may not be true).

Our interest in doing things and finding things encourages doctors to test. But the tests themselves have an appeal, particularly those that produce pictures. A lot of us are technophiles, and there is no place with more "way cool" technology than the radiology department of a major hospital.

The pictures that we have access to nowadays are great. All the information is digitized, meaning that computers can store and manipulate the images, which are then projected on large screens. Even a standard chest X-ray can be made lighter or darker, given more or less contrast, and have sections enlarged or reduced. And that's entry-level stuff. More advanced images get color enhanced, made to look 3-D, rotated in space, or sequenced to show motion. And it gets better every year.

Money

I'd be remiss if I didn't say something about money. Radiology departments and clinical labs have long been moneymakers for hospitals. Recently, however, private-practice doctors have become more likely to have a financial interest in testing. This may range from doing simple lab tests in the office to owning a free-standing imaging center. Needless to say, a conflict of interest may arise when the doctor who orders the test also stands to make money in the process.

The classic proof of this problem came about a decade ago in a study comparing physicians who used imaging equipment in their own office with physicians who sent their patients elsewhere to get X-rays.[3] The authors were careful to say they didn't know what the right amount of testing was, but they clearly concluded that owning the equipment influenced behavior: doctors with their own equipment ordered more than four times as many X-rays as doctors who sent their patients to outside providers.

Of course, it's not surprising that having a financial stake influences a physician's decisions about testing. You just need to be aware that that may be the case. For years primary care doctors have complained that procedural services—tests and surgeries—are much more lucrative than cognitive services—learning about you, listening to your problems, thinking about what is wrong, and proposing a reasonable course of action. The complaint is warranted. Many have responded, moreover, by developing "billable services"—which typically involve testing. So doctors buy kits to test blood, various pieces of fiber-optic equipment (sigmoidoscopes, colposcopes), treadmills, ultrasound units, and X-ray machines. And if they've got them, they tend to use them.

The opposite problem also exists: some doctors have a financial interest in *not* doing tests. The payment arrangement in some for-profit physician networks includes a so-called credit for primary care doctors whose referral rates for imaging tests (and specialists) are lower than average. Understandably, such an arrangement has received a lot of publicity and been severely criticized.

Everybody understands that financial incentives influence behavior. The worry we most often hear about is underservice. But overservice is a real problem too. I wish doctors didn't face financial incentives in testing in either direction. But many do, and because it matters, you should know about it.

Patients

One other force encourages doctors to test, and that is patients. Some patients see tests as more objective than their physicians (even though many tests, such as X-rays and biopsies, still involve humans making subjective determinations) and more likely to produce a definite answer in the event of a specific problem. Some want tests simply to reassure them that they are well—or to validate that they are sick. And as I said earlier, there is the widespread presumption that it never hurts to look. So even though not all patients in fact want to be tested, many doctors tend to assume that they do. If you feel differently, just letting your doctor know may make a big difference.

FORCES THAT INFLUENCE THE SYSTEM

To understand the medical culture, it's not enough to know about doctors. Increasingly, medical care delivery is influenced by "systems." The word *system,* though heard a lot in medicine these days, does not have a precise definition in this context. For simplicity, let's say it refers to the managerial structures in place to deliver medical care. The United States doesn't have one system, it has thousands of them. And while the managerial structures may differ, everyone has some sort of managed care, from charity care in county hospitals to the most generous fee-for-service insurance plans.

Health care managers who work for these systems frequently promote preventive testing, particularly testing for cancer. Some are undoubtedly motivated by the best intentions, truly believing that testing for cancer is in the population's best interest. But there are other, less altruistic, interests served by promoting cancer testing, which need to be taken into account as well.

Cancer testing as good public relations

Given the old adage that an ounce of prevention is worth a pound of cure, it is perhaps not surprising that preventive medicine is more or less universally endorsed. For the last 30 years or so, moreover, the medical system has been criticized for being more concerned with treating disease than preventing it.[4] Not only does the criticism make a good sound bite, but it is, of course, true.

Unfortunately, many people have gone on to conclude that doctors should focus on preventing disease instead of treating it. While this is a very appealing notion on the surface, the reality is more complex. True prevention (e.g., keeping adolescents from smoking or getting them in the habit of using seatbelts) is best accomplished in social settings other than a doctor's office. Physicians' preventive efforts are narrower, and largely involve looking for early forms of disease. Functionally, this means ordering tests—an exercise, as we have seen, with problems of its own.

Nevertheless, managers love to promote their system's preventive services. Preventing disease has broad public appeal because it both applies to so many people and has the luster of being a public health service. It is a tangible way of showing that their system "cares." Because cancer is such a scary disease, cancer prevention programs have special appeal. Breast and cervical cancer screening have the extra appeal of addressing women's health issues. In short, many managers see cancer testing as good PR.

Cancer testing as measurable quality improvement

The current effort to make medicine more systematic has served to promote cancer testing too. In the last decade, medical managers have looked to the manufacturing industry to help reduce error and to make the "product" of medicine more consistent from doctor to doctor. Quality improvement teams, which have sprung up in many health care organizations, strive to introduce "systems thinking" among health care providers. While these efforts can be useful, they are limited to those functions that can in fact be made systematic—such routine processes as preparing a patient for elective surgery or monitoring the use of blood thinners in patients prone to clotting, for instance—and whose output is measurable and in which "improvement" can be gauged—shorter waiting times, or having more patients whose blood is thinned within the desired range.

Cancer testing fits this scheme nicely. It is a routine service. It is easy to know whether it happens or not. And the goal is clear: to test more people. For these reasons, the rate of cancer testing is one of the most common quality measures appearing on health care report cards.[5]

Two things about this trend concern me. The first has to do with the (understandable) use of measures that are convenient. If systems focus on what they can easily measure, it is inevitable that they will miss an important part of health care. Managers like having a list of services that physicians should provide during an outpatient encounter. It helps define the product, makes it more measurable, and makes the physician more accountable. But even if the services are useful, these efforts can distract from more important issues—those most relevant to the sick, which get crowded out by those most relevant to the healthy.[6]

My second concern has to do with how physicians react to being measured. We all want to perform well; in fact, we were selected for medical school based on our good grades in college. If "getting a good grade" in medical practice means making sure that 100 percent of women we see get a mammogram or a Pap smear, that is what most of us will try to do—even if the women don't want to be tested. The desire to perform well may lead us, if not to outright coercion, at least to persuasive tactics: overstating the benefit, ignoring the downsides, and suggesting that people are making a mistake if they don't follow our recommendations.

Cancer testing as good business

For systems that are trying to attract new patients, especially people who might not otherwise seek health care, there is yet another benefit to promoting cancer testing. One of the best ways to identify potential patients is to aggressively screen a population for disease. Currently, breast cancer screening epitomizes this approach. "Breast care centers," set up by health care systems, both promote screening and coordinate all subsequent services: biopsy, lumpectomy, plastic surgery, chemotherapy, and radiation. The health care management literature is filled with articles on how to enhance their profitability.

Also benefiting from cancer screening and preventive medicine generally are the for-profit systems that insure patients. Think about it. For insurers, the most reliable way to make money is to cover those least likely to need services. And who cares most about screening for cancer and heart disease? Not patients who already have cancer or heart disease. The people attracted to these services are the people who *don't* have cancer or heart disease. Anyone who is sick is more concerned with a system's ability to care for the ill than with its preventive services.

FORCES INFLUENCING RESEARCHERS

Finally, there is one more part of the culture of medicine with which you should be familiar: the world of medical researchers. Because many medical researchers are also doctors, you might think of it as a subculture. But researchers are subject to some unique forces. Research also strongly influences the information you receive, both in the media and from doctors. It is therefore important to know something about how medical research works.

The first thing to know is that research is far from a wholly objective enterprise. Distortions can occur at any stage, ranging from blatant fabrication of data (rare but not unheard of), to convenient dismissal of data that do not agree with our beliefs (much more common), to the unintentional biases that creep in as we design our studies (undoubtedly a daily occurrence).

The second thing to know is that all researchers are interested in gaining attention. Traditionally, this has meant publishing in the scientific literature (following the familiar academic dictum "Publish or perish"). Increasingly, however, researchers have garnered attention via the popular media. Professional and public recognition is often a strong motivating force for us as we seek to present our findings.[7]

The final thing to know is that our publishing venues have interests of their own. The popular media are interested in good, simple stories; "medical breakthroughs" are both compelling and easy to explain. The scientific journals, interested in increasing their own profile in the media, typically send news releases to the media, leading to their articles being covered in popular magazines and newspapers. Even the universities and hospitals we work for, wanting good publicity themselves, may publicize or advertise the work of their researchers. Here the focus is on new and flashy technologies not widely available elsewhere. All of these groups are relatively uninterested in research that shows that some new test or treatment is no better than an old one.

You can guess the end result of these forces. Researchers get strongly vested in a particular test or treatment. (Some even have their salaries supported by manufacturers.) Research findings may be selectively reported: findings suggesting benefit are exaggerated, while those suggesting no benefit—or worse, harm—are minimized or not reported at all. The result is that most of what you hear in health news concerns only what is allegedly new and better.

I do not mean to suggest that all medical research is falsified or that most researchers are dishonest. There is a lot of good research—and many good researchers—out there. But in general, it is legitimate to say that medical research is biased in favor of new tests and treatments and that the findings of this work are frequently exaggerated. For you, this means that a certain amount of skepticism is always in order when evaluating medical news.

To be sure, some researchers, not tied to industry, seriously try to analyze what works and what doesn't in medicine. When the utility of a new test or treatment is ambiguous or the data weak, they make every effort to let practicing physicians know. When it comes to cancer screening, however, the opposing forces they face may be overwhelming.

Consider what happened in 1997 when the National Cancer Institute (NCI) tried to evaluate the use of mammography for women aged 40 to 50.[8] The director of the NCI convened a 13-member panel of impartial medical experts and consumer advocates and asked them to review all the data available on the subject. The goal was to provide some consensus recommendations for American women. This is the time-honored approach to difficult questions used by all the National Institutes of Health (of which the NCI is one); more than a hundred of these consensus panels have been assembled in the past.

The panel concluded that the evidence supporting mammography in this age group was weak. If it did save lives—which was far from clear to begin with—very few would benefit: less than one per 1,000 women screened for an entire decade. And there were clearly downsides: roughly a third of women would have at least one false positive exam, and a substantial number would be told they had cancer, and would be treated for cancer, when in fact they had pseudodisease, a cancer that would never cause symptoms.[9] All in all, the benefits of mammography were simply too close to call. So the panel came to the only reasonable conclusion possible: rather than issuing a yea or nay proclamation, they suggested that individual women should make their own choice.

The reaction to the panel's conclusion was anything but reasonable, and the behavior of a number of prominent academic physicians was decidedly unscholarly. Despite obvious self-interest, radiologists went straight to the news media:[10] one suggested the panel was condemning American women to death, another called the report fraudulent.[11] Bernadine Healy, the former head of the National Institutes of Health and a prominent supporter of women's health issues, stated that she was "very disturbed that a group of so-called experts challenged the notion of early detection"— even as she acknowledged that she had not read the report. The director of the NCI said he was "shocked" by the outcome, leading many to wonder why he convened the panel if he already knew there was a "right answer."

The politicians didn't behave much better. Senator Arlen Specter (R-Pa.) summoned the panel's chairman to defend the recommendation at a special hearing of the Senate Subcommittee on Labor, Health and Human Services, and Education Appropriations. The Senate went on to vote for a nonbinding resolution supporting mammography for women in their 40s. No one wanted to be on the wrong side of this issue: the vote was 98 to 0. The director of the NCI, now under considerable political pressure, asked his advisory board (a board established to advise the director on NCI policy) to review the panel's recommendation. At first they declined, not wanting to interfere with the time-honored process, but eventually they voted 17 to 1 in favor of recommending mammography to all women in their 40s.

This example highlights some of the forces that work to preclude rational discourse about research findings on cancer testing. There will always be an asymmetry among testing proponents and detractors. Testing proponents have a very strong interest (often financial) in promoting tests—much more so than the researchers trying to critically evaluate them. Proponents have powerful anecdotes, about individuals whose lives may have been "saved" because their cancer was caught early (if perhaps unnecessarily). And because those who commit their career to a particular test or treatment generally become proponents of that technology, proponents tend to wear the mantle of technical expertise. Detractors, in contrast, often evaluate multiple technologies, and so their expertise lies not in the ins and outs of the techniques in question, but in measuring their effect on patients.

SUMMARY

Much in the culture of medicine promotes cancer testing. Doctors are trained to look for disease and are rewarded, professionally and sometimes financially, when they find it. Testing is also seen as protection against malpractice suits. And doctors want to use new tests because they think patients expect them to.

Cancer testing is also promoted by other players in the system. Health care managers promote cancer testing because it's good public relations. For them, screening is an easily quantifiable measure of health care quality, and one that is easy to improve. Medical researchers frequently have interests in "proving" that new tests are better. Although the most common interest is professional recognition, increasingly financial interests are also present.

In order to be a better-informed consumer, therefore, you need to know that not all you hear about cancer testing is the unsullied truth. Some of the push for testing, to be sure, is due to "true believers"—those who believe that any effort to prevent cancer must be good and helpful. But a more complex, less idealistic set of forces is behind the push as well. Now that you understand the need for healthy skepticism in assessing the need for tests, you are ready to learn about the numbers we use to test the tests.

EIGHT

Understand the statistics of cancer (and why five-year survival is the world's most misleading number)

While this subject may sound intimidating, don't worry. If you are a little unsure exactly what the word *statistic* means, you are in good company. To be sure, I had to look it up in the dictionary. (For the record, a "statistic" is merely a number that is computed from a set of observations, the most familiar being a simple average.) I will only talk about three statistics, and each is basically a simple fraction—a numerator over a denominator.

And in case you are thinking that this subject will be boring, again I'll say: don't worry. In this chapter you will learn how easy it is to be misled by an apparently straightforward, unambiguous number. And you'll see that, whether they are interpreted correctly or not, these three statistics influence many important decisions.

Just as knowing something about prices, inventories, and consumer demand helps us understand various sectors of the economy, knowing something about cancer incidence, mortality, and five-year survival rates helps us understand various cancers. These are the vital signs of cancer. Incidence addresses the question "How frequently do people get this cancer?" Mortality (also known as a cancer death rate) addresses the question "How frequently do people die of it?" And five-year survival addresses the question most relevant to a newly diagnosed cancer patient: "Now that I have this cancer, how likely am I to be alive five years from now?"

Because these questions are of widespread interest, many people work hard to assemble the statistics that address them. Here in the United States, new cases of cancers from various regions in the country are carefully cataloged, including information on how widespread the disease is, what the cells look like, what treatment patients receive, how long they live, and why they die. The nationwide data have been consistently collected since 1973, and in the state of Connecticut since the 1950s. It is without question the best cancer cataloguing system in the world.

As you might imagine, these statistics have a tremendous influence on how we judge the need for cancer testing and how we judge its success. But what is less obvious is how these statistics could be collected so carefully and so well, yet still be so misleading—in large part *because* of cancer testing.

DEALING WITH THE UNEXPECTED

In Chapter 4 I told you about a patient who called me because he was hoarse and ended up being told he had kidney cancer. I purposely didn't finish the story then because what happened next is more relevant here.

This man, you will recall, had a small cancer on his vocal cords. It hadn't spread anywhere, and it was easily removed. But as part of his evaluation we got a chest X-ray, which raised the question of an abnormality in the chest, which led to a CAT scan of the chest, which showed that there wasn't any problem in the chest but raised questions about the kidney, which led to a CAT scan of the abdomen, which detected what was almost certainly a kidney cancer. It was a testing cascade that led to a totally unexpected finding.

The question was what to do next. I discussed the issue with a radiologist and a cancer surgeon. Both were convinced that this was cancer. Because the mass had pockets of fluid in between areas of tissue, neither thought a needle biopsy would be helpful; a negative biopsy would simply mean the needle had missed the tissue. So their advice was simple: take the kidney out.[1]

Neither the patient nor I felt very good about that. Sure, he had another kidney, and we had every reason to believe he could manage well with just one. But taking out a kidney is a serious operation: the incision is big, so he would be very sore for weeks afterward, and some people do die from the operation (for an average patient in his mid-60s, the expectation is about 12 deaths per 1,000 operations).[2] And most important, my patient felt well. He wasn't taking any medicines, he had stopped smoking three years earlier, he was walking over three miles a day, he regularly traveled to New York City to visit friends. Indeed, removing the vocal cord tumor had fixed the only thing that *was* bothering him: hoarseness. Why upset the apple cart?

The cancer surgeon was taken aback that I would even entertain such thinking. He thought I should be forcefully persuading the patient to aggressively fight this cancer. He looked at the same patient, saw the same person, and came to a totally different conclusion. His assessment was straightforward: "Look, here is an otherwise healthy guy who has kidney cancer. Yes, it's major surgery, but because he's healthy he'll sail through it. We've got the chance to save this man's life."

I hate being on the other side of this argument. Why would any doctor want to forgo the chance to save someone's life? But my patient and I shared a sense of unease about where we were—and how we had gotten there. Maybe it was a fast-growing cancer. Maybe it had just started growing. Maybe it hadn't yet begun to spread and surgery would solve the problem—that is, maybe we had stumbled on it at just the right time. But that would be incredibly good timing. In fact, the chances were much more likely it had been there a long time—that it was a slow-growing cancer. The patient wanted to know why we couldn't simply check on it again in another three months.

The cancer surgeon persisted, and now he had statistics. He told me that when we remove a kidney cancer before it metastasizes, 90 percent of patients are alive in five years. But if we wait until after it metastasizes, only 10 percent of patients are alive in five years. He went on to point out that because of early detection, the average five-year survival for patients with kidney cancer had increased from 34 percent in 1950 to 62 percent currently. Pretty convincing stuff.

I thought I ought to check his statistics.[3] He was right. Patients with early-stage kidney cancers are much more likely to survive five years than those whose cancers have spread beyond the kidney. Because of CAT scans, we are finding more kidney cancers at an earlier stage than we did in the past. Most important, the proportion of Americans with kidney cancer who are surviving five years is increasing. The evidence seemed conclusive: testing for cancer is helping people live longer.

But I noticed something else: the number of Americans *dying* from kidney cancer is not decreasing.

AN APPARENT PARADOX

The five-year survival rate is rising, but mortality is not falling. Both numbers are right. The question, in that case, is *Why* isn't kidney cancer mortality falling?

First, you might guess that the growth in the U.S. population explains why kidney cancer mortality hasn't fallen. This is perfectly plausible: as the country gets bigger, you would expect more people to die from cancer. But I oversimplified mortality above by referring to "the number of Americans dying." Rather, it is the annual rate at which people die. More precisely, for kidney cancer it is the number of Americans who die from kidney cancer every year divided by the total number of Americans that year. Stated as a fraction, it looks like this:

$$\frac{\text{number of deaths from kidney cancer per year}}{\text{total population}}$$

Mortality rates are usually expressed as the number of deaths per 100,000 people; the current mortality rate for kidney cancer, for example, is a little over 3 per 100,000.[4] The significant part of all this is that because the denominator is the *total* population, the mortality statistic is automatically corrected for changes in the size of that population.

Incidence—or how frequently people get a particular disease—looks a lot like mortality (and is also expressed as the number of cases per 100,000), except the numerator is different:

$$\frac{\text{number of new cases of kidney cancer per year}}{\text{total population}}$$

Five-year survival is a fundamentally different statistic from mortality and incidence. It tells what proportion of people with a particular cancer are alive five years after diagnosis. Thus, the denominator is not the population but the number of patients diagnosed with a certain cancer at a particular time. The numerator is the number of those patients who are alive five years later:

$$\frac{\text{number of patients alive 5 years after kidney cancer diagnosis}}{\text{number of patients diagnosed with kidney cancer}}$$

Now that I have more completely defined the statistics, lets get back to the question of why kidney cancer mortality isn't falling. You might suggest another explanation: although patients with kidney cancer are living to an older age, they still ultimately die from kidney cancer. Put another way, while real progress is being made in detecting and fighting kidney cancer (living to an older age being a sign of that), there is still no cure—and so mortality remains constant. Again, this is a perfectly plausible explanation, and again, I have oversimplified how mortality is measured. Mortality rates are adjusted for age; thus, if people with kidney cancer die at an older age now than in previous years, kidney cancer mortality will fall.[5] But that's not happening.

So again: why is five-year survival in kidney cancer rising while kidney cancer mortality remains steady? Rising five-year survival sounds like it should be good news. Curiously, this is one of the paradoxes in early cancer detection. The statistic is not telling you what you really want to know.

WHETHER IT BENEFITS PATIENTS OR NOT, CANCER TESTING INFLATES FIVE-YEAR SURVIVAL

There are two reasons why five-year survival might go up without any change in the cancer death rate. The first is that patients are being diagnosed with kidney cancer earlier in life, but they die at the same age. The second—and this is the kicker—is that some patients are diagnosed with kidney cancer who never would have been before. They have pseudo-disease: a cancer that was never destined to cause symptoms, much less kill them. But since we are not sure which patients have pseudodisease, all who are diagnosed with "cancer" are included in the calculation of five-year survival, which makes average survival appear to look better than it did before cancer testing became so widespread.

Of the three cancer statistics, five-year survival is the one you'll see and hear most commonly. It is also the one most likely to mislead. So it is important to fully understand the two explanations for how cancer testing can increase five-year survival without anyone benefiting.

Patients are diagnosed earlier in life but die at the same age

Think about measuring survival time. It's obvious when to stop the clock: when an individual dies. But when should you start the clock? In practice, the clock is started when an individual is found to have cancer—at the time of diagnosis. Of course, the cancer has been around before that, so "survival time" is only a portion of the true duration of the cancer:

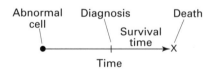

Patients with cancers detected by screening are diagnosed earlier in the course of their disease, before they develop symptoms: such is the nature of screening. Because they are diagnosed earlier, these patients will survive "longer" even if early treatment has no effect—because the length of survival is being measured *from the time of diagnosis*. Measuring survival time thus answers only this question: If my cancer is diagnosed with a test (instead of when symptoms appear), will I live longer from the time of diagnosis? The answer is yes. It doesn't, however, address the question you really want answered: If my cancer is diagnosed with a test, will I live to an older age? Here, the answer is "Not necessarily."

Think about two groups of patients who develop kidney cancer, one in the past (say 25 years ago), the other today. In the past, patients with kidney cancer were diagnosed because of some symptom, such as pain or bloody urine. Let's say all the men in our hypothetical group were diagnosed at the same age: 67 years old. Today, because of advanced imaging technologies, assume we find all of these cancers earlier in the disease course—age 60, say. But suppose that all the men in both groups die at age 70 (which is, in fact, the typical age of death for men with kidney cancer). Here's a simplified illustration of the comparison:

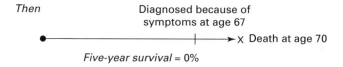

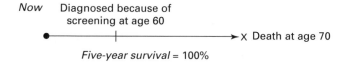

What's your assessment? I suspect you won't say that patients today are any better off. Indeed, you might argue that they are worse off, because they must live longer with the knowledge they have cancer. But you wouldn't know this from the five-year survival statistic, which in the past was 0 percent and now is 100 percent.

Of course, all kidney cancer patients are not diagnosed at the same age, nor do they all die at the same age. It would be more realistic in the above example to think of average survival time, which in a real-world sample of kidney cancer patients might be 3.2 years in the past versus 7.8 years now. Of course, buried in that 3.2-year average would be a few patients who survived five years, while the 7.8-year average would include a few patients who did not survive that long. In reality, then, five-year survival rates are always somewhere in between 0 percent and 100 percent. None of this should obscure the basic truth, however. Although we all tend to think, when we hear "longer survival" or "increased five-year survival," that death has been delayed, it is equally likely that diagnosis simply occurred earlier in life.

Some patients are diagnosed with cancers that do not progress

Not only is five-year survival affected by when we start the clock, it is also affected by which patients we select to track. In the past, when symptoms led to a cancer diagnosis, most people found to have cancer had an aggressive, fast-growing disease. Now, as more and more cancers are detected by screening, many who receive a cancer diagnosis have a more slowly progressing disease. And some have pseudodisease, a cancer that doesn't progress at all. Both these groups have essentially "watered down" the five-year survival statistic.

Suppose, by way of simplified illustration, that there are just two forms of kidney cancer: progressive and nonprogressive. In the past, only the progressive form was detected. Of 1,000 patients with progressive cancer, let's say that 400 lived five years. Today we find those same cancers, and the same number survive five years. But in addition, because of testing (in this case with abdominal CAT scans) we also find 1,000 patients with nonprogressive kidney cancer, all of whom are alive in five years. So now we have 2,000 cancer patients, 1,400 of whom are alive after five years. Figure 15 illustrates these changes.

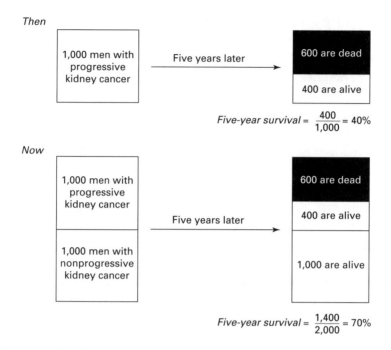

Figure 15.   How diagnosing nonprogressive cancer inflates five-year survival.

What's your assessment? Again, I'd be surprised if you said that patients today are better off. Indeed, you might argue that they are worse off, since some are being told unnecessarily that they have cancer. But you wouldn't know this from the five-year survival rate, which has apparently "improved" from 40 percent in the past to 70 percent now.

FAULTY COMPARISONS USING FIVE-YEAR SURVIVAL

Because five-year survival is affected by the *timing* of diagnosis and *who* is diagnosed, it is an unreliable statistic for drawing conclusions about the quality of medical care across time. But that doesn't stop people from making faulty comparisons based on five-year survival and promoting those comparisons as evidence of the value of cancer research and early detection.

In 1999, for example, former Vice President Gore, arguing against Republican tax cuts that would have resulted in a smaller budget for the National Institutes of Health, announced that five-year survival rates for all cancers had risen to almost 60 percent in the early 1990s, up from 51 percent in the early 1980s.[6] In reality, however, the mortality rate for all cancers combined *increased* over that period (although they have gone down since then). Similarly, in 1998 Senator Kay Bailey Hutchinson (R-Tex.) made the case for breast cancer screening on the floor of the U.S. Senate: "When detected early and when confined to the breast, the 5-year survival rate for this disease is over 95%. Mr. President, this is a remarkable statistic, and represents a dramatically improved picture than [*sic*] that of even a few years ago."[7] Yet as the next chapter shows, there is considerable debate about whether mammography really *does* work.

Faulty comparisons are also made between countries. The Office of National Statistics in the United Kingdom noted that five-year survival for colon cancer was 60 percent in the United States compared to 35 percent in Britain. British experts reacted to the finding as "disgraceful," and many called for a doubling of government spending on cancer treatment. In response, Prime Minister Tony Blair vowed to increase survival rates by 20 percent over the next 10 years, decrying the fact that "we don't match other countries in its [colon cancer's] prevention, diagnosis and treatment."[8] In fact, despite the gap in five-year survival rate statistics, the mortality rate for colon cancer in England is only slightly higher than that in the United States. The comparison is even more faulty for prostate cancer. In the early 1990s, the prostate cancer five-year survival rate was a little over 40 percent in the United Kingdom, versus over 90 percent in the United States. While it might be tempting to conclude that our medical care system is vastly superior, the U.S. mortality rate at the time was actually slightly higher than the British rate. Our prostate cancer five-year survival is so much higher only because we tell so many more people they have prostate cancer.

I don't want to be misunderstood, so let me be very clear about what I am not saying and what I am saying.

What I am not saying

1. I'm not saying that rising five-year survival rates are never good news. Just because cancer testing—which leads to earlier diagnosis and the increased likelihood of finding nonprogressive cancers—will always increase five-year survival, it doesn't mean that rising five-year survival is always only an artifact of cancer testing. Increased five-year survival may reflect one or two pieces of "good news." First, new cancer treatments may be genuinely more effective than old ones. Second, old treatments may simply be more effective when we begin them earlier (thanks to cancer testing).

But for either of these pieces of "good news" to be true, cancer mortality should drop. We have seen this happen, most dramatically in testicular cancer, and we may be beginning to see it in breast and colon cancer. The bottom line is that meaningful improvements in detection or treatment ought to affect not just five-year survival but also mortality.

2. I'm not saying that five-year survival is always an ambiguous statistic. In a randomized trial of two cancer treatments, the treatment producing the longer five-year survival is without doubt more effective. Here's how a randomized trial of therapy works: Newly diagnosed cancer patients are invited to join the study. Those who agree are randomly assigned one of two treatments. The five-year survival clock starts at the same time in both groups: at the time of enrollment. Because the two groups are essentially the same except for treatment received and because the clock starts at the same time, we can be confident that the group with the higher five-year survival rate did in fact put off death. So five-year survival is a perfectly valid measure in a randomized trial of cancer (or any other) therapy.[9]

What I am saying

Cancer testing has a powerful effect on five-year survival rates. Individuals diagnosed with different diagnostic tests and at different times in the course of their disease should always be expected to have different five-

year survival rates. Expect higher five-year survival rates in patients diagnosed with new, more sensitive tests and lower ones in patients diagnosed with old tests. Expect higher five-year survival rates in patients with
early-stage cancer and lower ones in patients with late-stage cancer. And
because every year we find cancers earlier, expect that five-year survival
rates will continue to increase over time, for all cancers.[10]

None of this, however, tells you anything about the usefulness of cancer testing (or the usefulness of treatment). For that you have to look elsewhere. Surprisingly, a fair number of doctors don't understand the problems associated with five-year survival rates. And I am sorry to report
that some of them do research, research that gets published in the medical literature and even reported in the general press. Here's an example,
from the *Toronto Star:*

> The Boston study compared the outcomes for 117 women age 40 to 49
> whose breast cancer was diagnosed by mammography with that of 928
> women whose cancer was detected by physical examination. It found
> that 40 per cent of the women whose cancers were diagnosed by mam-
> mography had precancerous tumors that had not spread into surround-
> ing tissue while only 9 per cent of women in the physician exam group
> had this very early type of tumor. The five-year survival rate for women
> whose tumor was found by mammography was 96 per cent compared
> with 74 per cent for patients in the other group.[11]

Now you know what this does and does not tell you. It tells you that
mammography finds smaller cancers than a physical exam. You expect that.
It tells you that women whose cancers were diagnosed by mammography
were more likely to be alive five years after diagnosis than women whose
cancer was diagnosed by physical exam. You expect that too. It doesn't tell
you whether finding cancer early delayed anyone's death. It also doesn't
tell you something else that is very important: Were all the cancers diagnosed by mammography destined to become a problem?

I can pretty much guarantee that you'll see the same basic argument
again and again—maybe involving a different test and a different cancer,
but the pattern is predictable. Step 1 is to use a cancer test to find early-
stage cancers. Step 2 is to observe that the test does what it is supposed

to do: find patients whose cancers are at earlier stages than patients whose cancer was found without the test. Step 3 is to observe that patients whose cancer was found by the test have a higher five-year survival rate. Step 4 is to call for screening using the test.

This pattern has recently appeared in the medical literature, with UCLA researchers calling for kidney cancer screening and Cornell researchers calling for lung cancer screening.[12] The Cornell findings quickly made it to the *New York Times,* where one of the researchers was quoted as saying, "The method [spiral CAT scans] could allow as many as 80 percent of lung cancer patients to survive at least five years. Just 15 percent live that long now."[13] What she didn't mention was what you learned in Chapter 4: spiral CAT scan technology turns up about 10 times as many lung cancer cases as do chest X-rays, and finds almost as many lung cancers in nonsmokers as in smokers.[14] In other words, it finds a lot of lung cancer we never knew existed.

I'm afraid that the bottom line is this: When you hear the term *five-year survival,* you need to be suspicious. If it appears in the context of a randomized trial of cancer therapy, you can be confident that the measure is valid. But if the term is juxtaposed with a cancer test or the words *early diagnosis* or *screening,* alarms should go off. Either someone is trying to persuade you with a comparison they know is faulty or they really don't know what they are talking about.

CANCER TESTING INFLATES INCIDENCE

Incidence—the rate at which new cases are diagnosed—is an important statistic as well. If different countries have different incidence rates, most observers conclude that there are real differences in the underlying frequency of the cancer, which may help us learn more about why people get cancer. And if incidence is rising in a country, many will also conclude that morbidity (harmful effects other than death) and mortality from cancer are destined to go up. Occasionally someone will even use a frightening term: cancer epidemic.

Let's return to kidney cancer and consider what is happening to its incidence. It's rising: the age-adjusted rate is more than double what it was 50 years ago. Is there an epidemic of kidney cancer? In a word: no. I don't know anyone who believes that all of the rising incidence is real—that is, that people are truly developing kidney cancer at twice the rate of 1950. Instead most, if not all, of the increased incidence is the result of doctors finding kidney cancer more often.

In a perfect world, testing for cancer wouldn't influence how many patients are diagnosed, it would only influence when they are diagnosed. In reality, however, testing can dramatically influence the cancer incidence rate (see appendix at the end of this chapter).

This phenomenon undoubtedly explains the increased incidence observed in cancers of organs deep inside the body. These organs are in places we couldn't see using conventional X-rays. Then came ultrasounds, CAT scans, MRIs, and the ability to direct skinny needles into these organs to perform biopsies. The result is that since 1950 a number of "epidemics" have seemed to appear. The incidence of cancers of the brain is up 70 percent, kidney cancer up 130 percent, liver cancer up 180 percent, and prostate cancer up 195 percent—almost three times the incidence in 1950.[15] The word *epidemic* has been most frequently used to describe the cancer incidence for a more accessible organ: the breast. Part of the 65 percent increase in breast cancer incidence is also the result of testing—more women undergoing ever more sensitive mammograms.[16]

Oddly enough, the effect of testing on incidence is most dramatic for a cancer in an organ that sees the light of day: the skin. The cancer is melanoma, and it arises from the skin cells that produce pigment. Its incidence is up 477 percent, almost six times what it was in 1950. Most of the increase has been in early-stage cancers, ones less than 1.5 mm thick. While some of this increase may be the result of increased exposure to the sun, most of it is probably related to increased exposure to dermatologists.[17]

Their cancer test is a skin biopsy. In the past, a skin biopsy involved minor surgery. The skin was cleansed, covered with drapes, and injected with an anesthetic; then the doctor would use a scalpel to carefully cut away an ellipse of skin (a shape having a better cosmetic result). The hole would be closed with a few stitches, and the patient would come back a few days later to have them removed. Now a skin biopsy is typically done with a punch—a tool roughly the size of a pencil with a circular blade on the end. The punch takes a little circle of skin about this big: ● The hole gets one stitch or is sometimes just covered with a Band-Aid. Less pain, less work, less tissue, less time—and that equals more biopsies.

Furthermore, all doctors have been sensitized to look for melanoma. As a medical student, I remember a campaign to have us look thoroughly at all the skin of all patients. We were given little pocket cards reminding us what to look for. Patients with any suspicious moles were to be sent to dermatologists. That is how we screen for skin cancer, and it's been going on in doctors' offices for years. But it's getting more common. And you can imagine the chain of events: more people are referred to dermatologists,[18] more people get biopsied, more people are diagnosed with melanoma—and the incidence rate goes up.

A MELANOMA OUTBREAK

Rising incidence rates can get pretty scary. One of the classic examples occurred during the 1970s and '80s at Lawrence Livermore National Laboratory, across the bay from San Francisco. This lab is part of the U.S. Department of Energy and is engaged in nuclear weapons research as well as experimenting with various forms of energy. This is big-time physics and chemistry, so as you might imagine, there are potential exposures to all sorts of radiation and toxic substances.

In the mid-1970s a number of Livermore employees were diagnosed with melanoma. Although no known occupational exposures were associated with melanoma, California health officials—and presumably laboratory employees—were worried. They found that the incidence among Livermore employees was three times that of the surrounding community.

Investigators tried to nail down what was going on.[19] They compared the 19 employees who had been diagnosed with melanoma with those who had not. Employees with melanoma were no more likely to be scientists; they were no more likely to have been exposed to any type of radiation; they were no more likely to have worked in the lab a long time—in fact, their average tenure at Livermore was slightly less than that of workers who did not have melanoma. Adding to the mystery, there was no excess incidence of melanoma at the sister facility, Los Alamos National Laboratory in New Mexico, which hosted virtually identical research activities.

The story made it to the *New York Times* and the *Washington Post*. The incidence rate among laboratory employees continued to be more than twice that of neighboring counties through the early 1980s. But then investigators noticed something interesting: all the increase in incidence was in melanomas less than 1.5 millimeters thick—so-called thin melanoma. This is just the kind of small abnormality in which pseudodisease is bound to be common and about which pathologists are bound to disagree whether cancer is present. Investigators found no increase in the incidence of thick melanomas, however, and, more important, no increase in melanoma mortality among lab workers. And they noticed something else: laboratory employees were more likely to see dermatologists and more likely to have skin biopsies than others living in the same community. The difference was most dramatic after the initial reports of excess incidence, when employees were biopsied at nearly five times the rate of other people in the area.

What happened at Livermore? My guess is that the process was started by a chance event. All it would take is one staff member developing a very aggressive melanoma, due simply to bad luck, which quickly spreads and leads to death. Given preexisting concerns about a variety of exposures in the laboratory, coworkers become uneasy. Their response is understandable: they see a doctor and get checked for questionable moles. Questionable moles are of course found, and more skin biopsies are performed. Another case of melanoma is diagnosed. Concern spreads throughout the laboratory, and administrators feel pressed to respond. One tactic was in fact an "educational and awareness campaign," conducted by the laboratory's health services.

I also suspect that the involvement of the health department (and the press) began to influence the practice of local doctors, who examined Livermore employees more carefully and were more likely to biopsy. The patients looked harder, the doctors looked harder, there were more biopsies, and more early-stage melanoma was found.

The sad thing is that the worry seems to persist, affecting another generation. Just a few years ago, the *Los Angeles Times* reported on the high incidence of melanoma among children born in the area around the lab.

Over 30 years there had been eight cases, six more than statistically expected. But there had been no increase in the childhood cancers we know are related to radiation: leukemia and lymphoma.[20]

The natural response to concerns about a "cancer epidemic" is to look hard for cancer. Unfortunately, looking hard for cancer can be the cause of a cancer epidemic.

A CYCLE THAT ENCOURAGES TESTING

Rising incidence can create a positive feedback loop: it is both a *result of* and an *incentive for* more cancer testing. The same is true for rising five-year survival. The two combine to create a cycle of increasing aggressiveness in the search for cancer. The cycle looks something like this:

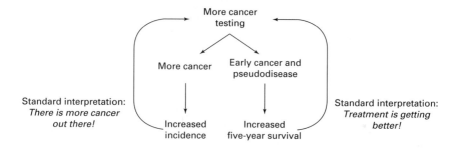

Here's how it plays out: a new test is developed, or an old one is done more frequently. More cancer is found. Incidence goes up. Someone uses the word *epidemic*. More testing is recommended. At the same time, cases of cancer are found earlier. Some are pseudodisease. Five-year survival rises. Someone uses the phrase *Saves lives*. More testing is recommended.

DOES CANCER TESTING REDUCE MORTALITY?

As I suggested earlier, the real question is, Does cancer testing reduce the rate at which people die from cancer? And the truth is, that can be hard to know.

Let me begin by saying that there is good news on the cancer front. Since 1950 mortality has fallen by more than half for cancers of the stomach, cervix, uterus, testis, and Hodgkin's disease, a cancer of the lymph glands.[21] And the mortality for cancers in children is a third of what it was 50 years ago. There is no ambiguity about how to interpret these dramatic declines. They are really good news.

But it's hard to know *why* cancer mortality has fallen. Too often the assumption is that declining mortality is due to cancer testing. In point of fact, though, a number of explanations are possible. The first may have nothing to do with medical care at all: reduced exposure to cancer-causing agents. Declining use of certain food preservatives, for example, is the explanation given by most experts for the fall in stomach cancer mortality. The second has everything to do with medical care but nothing to do with earlier detection: we have gotten better at treating cancer when it first causes symptoms. This is the predominant explanation for falling mortality in the cancers of childhood, Hodgkin's disease, and testicular cancer. The third has to do with earlier detection but has nothing to do with testing: patients with symptoms are increasingly aware of the importance of seeking care sooner rather than later. Older women's recognition that vaginal bleeding is abnormal after menopause, for example, may help explain the decline in uterine cancer. The final explanation is cancer testing: testing finds small, asymptomatic cancers that were destined to kill, cancers that are treatable at the time of testing but not after symptoms appear. Cancer testing, specifically the Pap smear, is the standard explanation given for the fall in cervical cancer—although other factors, such as improved hygiene generally and less sexually transmitted disease, undoubtedly play a role as well. (In addition, much of the value of the Pap smear may have less to do with pathologists—or more precisely, cytologists—examining cells under a microscope than with doctors actually seeing the cervix.)

Mortality for some other cancers is falling as well, if less dramatically. Since 1950 mortality from head and neck cancer, thyroid cancer, and bladder cancer are all down.[22] Although some environmental reasons may apply, my guess is that these declines are best explained by a combination of two factors: people with symptoms are seeking care earlier, and better treatment is available. Cancer testing is not a viable explanation, as no systematic testing exists for these cancers. Then there is colon and breast cancer, for which mortality is down by 25 percent and 15 percent, respectively. In both cases a systematic effort is being made to detect early disease. Are these two examples of where testing is really helping?

To be perfectly honest, it's hard to know. Most doctors (myself included) believe that a myriad of tests—fecal occult blood test, sigmoidoscopy, barium enemas, and colonoscopy—really are helping to reduce deaths from colon cancer. And the incidence of colon cancer is up only slightly, which means testing doesn't detect a lot of pseudodisease. Still, colon cancer testing does have problems, most notably excessive repetitive testing—annual colonoscopies following the detection of one or two polyps, for example.

Why there has been a small, but real, decline in breast cancer mortality is one of the hottest topics in medicine. Treatment really improved with the advent of hormonal therapy. And there is no doubt that women have become increasingly aware of the importance of having new lumps evaluated, often with a diagnostic mammogram. The usefulness of performing screening mammograms, however—that is, on women who do not have lumps—is a complicated subject, and the question of whether finding breast cancers that are too small to be felt hurts more than it helps remains open to debate. (See Chapter 9 for a full discussion.)

Then there is the not so good news. Prostate and ovarian cancer mortality remain essentially unchanged over the past 50 years, while mortality is rising for cancers of the esophagus, liver, pancreas, kidney, and brain as well as for melanoma. Finally, the worst news: in the last 50 years, the rate at which people die from lung cancer is up more than threefold. The explanation for this last increase can be summed up in a single word: smoking.

As I hope this chapter makes clear, of the three major cancer statistics—five-year survival, incidence, and mortality—mortality is the most important. It is simply the best statistic for making judgments about how well we are doing in controlling cancer. And it is the least subject to spurious influence of new cancer testing that inflates both incidence and five-year survival. Simply put: it is much easier to be certain about who dies of cancer than it is to be certain about who really has the disease and when it actually starts.

But even mortality can be problematic. Although there is no ambiguity about which people die and when, there is some ambiguity about *why* they die. First, simply knowing that a person has cancer influences how doctors determine the cause of death. So by finding more cancer, cancer testing may indirectly inflate apparent cancer mortality. Ironically, testing is likely responsible for much of the rising mortality of cancers we just couldn't "see" 50 years ago: cancer of the esophagus, liver, pancreas, kidney, and brain.

Then there's the question of what counts as a cancer death. If we are really interested in capturing true progress in cancer, cancer mortality should include not only deaths from cancer but also deaths from cancer treatment. In fact, ideally any deaths that occurred as a consequence of looking for cancer should be included as well. Consider an imaginary population with 500 deaths per 100,000 from cancer, with no early detection or treatment program in place. A few years later the death rate is 400 from the cancer, 40 from surgery for the cancer, 60 from chemotherapy/radiation, and 10 from the testing and biopsy process. Would you say there has been progress? I doubt it.

Most deaths during or immediately following cancer surgery do get counted in cancer mortality, but not all.[23] It is much more difficult to know whether chemotherapy and radiation deaths are being properly counted (and to be fair, it is very hard to do). And no one is keeping track of the deaths, however few, that are a consequence of the testing process. So even with our best statistic, there is room for improvement.

SUMMARY

Three fractions dominate how cancer is measured. Two are consistently influenced by cancer testing. Incidence rates may climb dramatically as more powerful diagnostic tools are developed and are used more frequently. Five-year survival—by far the most widely quoted cancer statistic, and the one most often used to promote the value of cancer testing—will likely also soar. This is the one you need to think most carefully about.

You need to remember that five-year survival will increase with time— even if not a single life is saved. Five-year survival can increase simply because we are telling people they have cancer earlier in their life (though their time of death does not change) and because we are telling more people they have cancer—that is, finding more pseudodisease. You should expect that new diagnostic tests and aggressive screening programs will always lead to increased five-year survival rates, even if early diagnosis doesn't help people live one day longer.

You should never accept five-year survival rates as evidence of the value of early cancer detection. They simply aren't valid estimates of whether cancer testing helps anybody. That's why carefully done research focuses on mortality rates. But there are limits to how much we can learn from even the best research, as I'll discuss in the next chapter.

APPENDIX: SPECIAL TOPICS

How age adjustment works

The three cancer statistics discussed in this chapter are always adjusted for age. The most important rationale for the adjustment is to make comparisons across years "fair" in the face of an aging population (to compare prostate cancer mortality in 1970, say, with prostate cancer mortality in 2003). Because older people are more likely to both get and die from virtually all adult cancers, without age adjustment incidence and mortality rates would continue to rise as the population ages. Health officials, however, want to distinguish changes in the frequency of cancer independent of the effects of an aging population.

Age adjustment helps do this. For convenience, I'll just talk in terms of mortality here, though the adjustment is exactly the same for incidence. First, mortality rates for the year of interest are calculated for each five-year age group (e.g., 30–34, 35–39). The result is 10 to 15 so-called age-specific rates (the exact number depends on how the very young and very old are grouped). To arrive at a single number, a summary rate is calculated: that is, a weighted average of the age-specific rates. The "weight" each age-specific rate gets depends on how many people were in the age group in 2000 (the so-called standard population). So a mortality statistic from one year—let's say 1970—is made comparable to another—

let's say 2003—by applying the same weights obtained for the 2000 population standard. Thus, if 5 percent of the 2000 population is age 30–34, then 5 percent of the 1970 mortality rate comes from 30–40-year-olds, as does 5 percent of the 2003 rate. An age-adjusted rate can thus be interpreted as what the 1970 (or 2003) death rate would have been if the population age distribution was exactly what it was in 2000.

Note that if cancer patients live longer, mortality will fall even if they still die of cancer. That is because the older age groups are smaller (i.e., there are fewer 80–84-year-olds than 75–79-year-olds), and they receive increasingly less weight in the summary rate. So delaying death to an older age has the effect of lowering the mortality rate (as it should).

In the case of five-year survival, cancer epidemiologists don't talk about age adjustment as such. Instead they talk about a "five-year relative survival rate." The fundamental motivation is the same, however. Consider the following: the typical age of a newly diagnosed prostate cancer patient is 70 years, that of a newly diagnosed testicular cancer patient is 33 years. Without knowing anything about the cancers, you can guess which cancer will probably have the higher five-year survival rate simply because younger people are more likely to live five more years than 70-year-olds are. The "relative" survival rate thus adjusts for the effect of age by comparing observed survival for patients with cancer to that expected in similar-aged people without cancer.

For example, the observed five-year survival rate for men with prostate cancer is 75 percent. But remember, most of these men are older and many die from other diseases, not prostate cancer. The expected five-year survival rate in men the same age without prostate cancer (the "general" population) is 78 percent. The five-year relative survival rate is the ratio of the two: 75 percent/78 percent, or 96 percent. The five-year relative survival rate is thus the proportion alive five years later relative to what would be expected in the general population. Because five-year survival in the average person is always lower than 100 percent, the five-year survival rate actually observed will always be lower than the relative survival that is reported. The effect of this is trivial in the young, but large in the elderly.

How testing inflates incidence rates

Cancer testing increases incidence rates even if the underlying amount of cancer is stable. There are two reasons for this. The first is easy to understand: testing detects pseudodisease. The cancer—which will never produce symptoms—has always been there, but thanks to more frequent testing it is being discovered more often. So incidence rates go up.

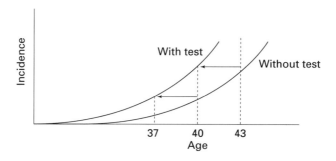

Figure 16. How early diagnosis increases age-adjusted incidence.

The second is an artifact of age adjustment, and a little tougher to understand. For most cancers, incidence rises with age: the older you are, the more likely you are to get cancer. In fact, as depicted in Figure 16, the rise is exponential. So simply advancing the time of diagnosis a few years has the effect of increasing the incidence rate for any given age group. If diagnosis is advanced three years, for example, what was the incidence rate for 40-year-olds becomes the incidence rate for 37-year-olds. The 40-year-olds now experience what was the incidence rate for 43-year-olds. And so on. It is as if you were shifting the incidence curve to the left. And because age-adjusted incidence is simply the weighted average of all the age-specific rates, it goes up too.

NINE   *Understand the limits to research—even*
genetic research (and why it is hard to be
sure there really are benefits to screening)

Helping other doctors learn how to do research is a big part of my job. As my mentor did for me, I pass on the cardinal rule of research: "If it's not published, it never happened." But writing is hard for most people. Luckily, there is a formulaic approach to writing a research report. First comes a section on what is known and why the research question is being addressed. Next, in the methods section, the researcher describes his or her research strategy. Then the main findings are presented, followed by a discussion of the findings and their limitations. Finally, there is a conclusion.

The conclusion can be tricky. That is the "sound bite" that will be communicated to doctors in practice—and in some cases, to the general public. So one wants to get it right. But what do the research findings really mean? What really should happen next? Good researchers are frequently hesitant to suggest major actions based on their findings. Not only are we trained to be cautious, but we also know the weaknesses of research better than most. In addition, we are fearful of being criticized by others in the research community. So we tend to avoid advocating a specific course of action, instead falling back on a well-worn conclusion: more research is needed.

I know, it's pretty pathetic. While this conclusion may be immune to criticism from other researchers, it also reeks of self-interest. What better way to conclude than by suggesting that there is more work for you and your colleagues to be paid to do? But there is another, less cynical way to think about this conclusion. It really represents a fundamental belief: that ultimately, the solution to any problem can be found through research. All we need is more.

But there are limits to what can be learned from research. And as you'll see in this chapter, nowhere is this more true than in research that examines the value of testing healthy people—people who have no symptoms of cancer—for early cancers. While it is relatively easy to learn whether a treatment helps sick patients, it is very difficult to learn whether testing can help those who are currently healthy. Hopes that the whole process will suddenly become more definitive as we learn to read our genes are overly optimistic.

TESTING THE TEST FOR BREAST CANCER

Let's begin with a deceptively simple question: Do mammograms work? Obviously, to answer this question someone has to decide what counts as "working." At one end of the spectrum, the question might be: Do mammograms find small cancers? At the other end of the spectrum the question would be: Does undergoing regular mammography lower a woman's overall chance of death (e.g., dying in the next 10 years)? Although I'll argue that this last question is the most relevant (and the one that patients hope doctors can give the answer to), let's focus on the slightly narrower question that the major studies have focused on: Does undergoing regular mammography lower the chance of death from breast cancer?

As I mentioned in Chapter 1, the first effort to answer this question began over 40 years ago. In the early 1960s, the Health Insurance Plan of Greater New York carried out the first randomized trial of mammography, known today as the HIP study. Because all the mammography studies I'm going to discuss are randomized trials, I need to review exactly what that means.

In its simplest form, a randomized trial is an experiment in which participants are assigned to one of two groups—e.g., mammography versus no mammography—solely by chance. (Although the approach is essentially like flipping a coin, the groups are in fact determined on the basis of random numbers generated by a computer.)[1] One group undergoes the "intervention"—the therapy or test being studied, in this case mammography. The other group, called the control group, does not—no mammography.

Randomization is the best way to construct two groups of subjects that are similar in every way except one—whether or not they are exposed to the intervention. Thus, groups selected at random are similar not only with respect to factors we know put people at risk for breast cancer death (e.g., age, menstrual history, family history of breast cancer), but also with respect to factors we have yet to learn about (e.g., the yet-to-be-discovered "cancer promoter gene" on chromosome 13). This means that any differences observed after the study has begun must be the *result* of the intervention. A randomized trial, in short, is the only way to be sure that a screening test works.

Good news

In the HIP study, 62,000 women were selected from the health plan patient list and were randomized into one of two groups by investigators. (The women were never aware of the randomization.) The intervention group was invited to have annual clinical breast exams—usually performed by a surgeon—and annual mammograms. The control group remained unaware that they were part of a study and continued to receive their usual medical care (at the time, no annual clinical exam and no mammogram). After 10 years of follow-up, the breast cancer death rate in the intervention group was 23 percent lower than that in the control group.[2]

Almost everybody assumes that this reduction was due to mammography. So as not to raise too many topics at once, I implied the same in Chapter 1. But as you can see from the design, the study really tested the combined effect of the clinical exam *and* mammography; indeed, it is impossible to discern the independent effect of either. It could be that mammography saved all the lives and the clinical exam added nothing, or the reverse could be true. No one can tell. All we can say is that women receiving the clinical breast exam and mammography did better than women receiving standard 1960s medical care, in which the breast was largely ignored.

In 1979, 45,000 women entered a trial in Edinburgh, Scotland, that, like the HIP study, evaluated the effectiveness of mammography plus clinical exam versus usual care. Unfortunately, instead of randomizing the 45,000 women, the researchers randomized the 84 general practices that cared for them. This failed to produce equivalent groups of women. Women in the control group were poorer and 20 percent more likely to die from reasons other than breast cancer. After seven years of follow-up, women cared for in practices that provided clinical exams and mammograms were reportedly 17 percent less likely to die from breast cancer.[3] However, because the women were so different otherwise, one could argue that the true effect of these screenings was considerably smaller or considerably larger. In the end, all we can say is that clinical breast exam and mammography *might* be better than the standard medical care. Given these uncertainties, I won't consider the Edinburgh study further.

At just about the same time, four randomized trials of mammography involving 280,000 women were carried out in Sweden: one in two rural provinces and the other three in the cities of Stockholm, Malmö, and Göteborg. As in the HIP study, women were unaware of their inclusion in a randomized trial. The intervention group was invited to undergo mammography (every 18 to 33 months); the other group continued usual medical care. After five to 13 years of follow-up, women in the mammography group had a 24 percent reduction in the breast cancer death rate.[4]

This time there was no confusion: it was mammography versus nothing. The sound bite was clear. "Mammography works."

Bad news

And then the Canadian study came along. Its sound bite was "No, it doesn't." In the world of cancer testing, no study has been so vigorously criticized. Before I tell you why, let me tell you what the Canadians did and what they found.

The Canadian National Breast Screening Study was the first of these trials to involve volunteers. All the women knew they were being studied and knew that they would be assigned to one of two groups by chance. This is important, because it is certainly plausible that these women were particularly motivated to find early breast cancers, so much so that they volunteered to be in the study—a factor that may help explain the results. The study really had two components: one for younger women and one for older women. Canada 1 randomized 50,000 women ages 40–49; one group received annual mammography and clinical breast exam, while the second received usual medical care. Canada 2 randomized 40,000 women ages 50–59, with one group receiving annual mammography and clinical breast exam, and the second receiving just the annual clinical breast exam. So Canada 1 was testing the effect of clinical breast exam and mammography in women in their 40s, while Canada 2 was testing the effect of *adding* mammography to clinical breast exam in women in their 50s. After seven years, both studies showed that women who received mammography had no reduction in breast cancer mortality.[5]

For screening proponents and mammographers, this finding was heretical—and their reaction was swift: the study was roundly condemned. The critique boiled down to two major allegations: (1) the mammography groups included a higher percentage of higher-risk women, making the comparisons unfair; and (2) the mammograms—and those who read them—were inadequate.

The unfair comparison criticism arose because it was alleged that as women entered the trial, study nurses directed women with a high risk of breast cancer to the mammography group.[6] In other words, the allegation was that the trial wasn't really randomized because women weren't assigned to groups solely by chance. The charge was taken very seriously, and Canada's National Cancer Institute ordered a review of the entire randomization process.[7] Two years later, the independent review was published; no credible evidence of subversion was found.[8] The heretical findings, therefore, could not be attributed to unfair comparison groups.

The allegation about inadequate mammography was twofold. First, the machines were said not to be "state of the art." Second, the radiologists or technologists were said to be insufficiently trained. Inferior machines, inferior professional personnel . . . as you might imagine, it was an American, not a Canadian, leading the charge.[9] The charge was an odd one, however. The American study of mammography conducted 20 years earlier, the HIP, certainly didn't have modern-day mammograms, yet proponents were happy to argue that it demonstrated mammography worked. More important, there is little doubt that the Canadian mammograms did what they were supposed to, which was find small cancers. More cancers were found in the women who received mammograms, and the cancers found were smaller than in control patients. In fact, the Canadian mammographers found more cancers and smaller cancers than did the mammographers in the Swedish studies.[10]

Reconciling the findings

So what was going on in Canada? From the perspective of readers of the scientific literature at least, these were the most carefully conducted randomized trials of mammography. And the reporting was meticulous: the randomization process, the comparability of the characteristics of women in the control and intervention group, the diagnostic procedures performed, how different cancers were found, the number of lymph nodes involved, the process used to determine cause of death, and the causes of death themselves were all described in detail. In fact, the level of detail reported undoubtedly increased the opportunity for criticism (there being more methodologic details to raise questions about).

In the context of what was known about breast cancer screening, were the findings really so heretical? Not especially. Let's look at all the randomized trials I've discussed, starting with the best-studied age group: women age 50 to 70. Think about what is being compared to what.

	Intervention group	Control group	Finding	Conclusion
HIP	clinical breast exam plus mammography	nothing	intervention better	some sort of breast exam is better than nothing
Swedish trials	mammography	nothing	intervention better	mammography is better than nothing
Canada 2	clinical breast exam plus mammography	clinical breast exam	no difference	mammography doesn't add to a *really* well done clinical breast exam

The HIP study compared clinical breast exam plus mammography to no screening and found that doing something was better than doing nothing. The four Swedish trials compared mammography to no screening and found that mammography was better than doing nothing. The Canadians compared clinical breast exam plus mammography to clinical breast exam and found that mammography didn't add anything. There's nothing inconsistent in these findings. All are perfectly plausible.

Now how about Canada 1 and women in their 40s? There it was mammography versus no screening—and the finding was that mammography was no better than doing nothing. Are there reasons mammography might not work in younger women? Probably. Younger women tend to have more aggressive cancers. Because they grow fast, they often become palpable during the interval between mammograms, rendering the mammogram useless. Furthermore, everyone agrees that it is harder to interpret mammograms in women with denser breasts, a condition more common in younger women.

But something else is different about younger women: they are less likely to get breast cancer—and they are less likely to die of it. That's good for the women, but a challenge for researchers trying to figure out whether screening works for younger women. Of the 50,000 women age 40 to 49 followed for seven years in Canada 1, for example, only 64 died of breast cancer. Not to sound crass, but that's not a lot of deaths for researchers to work with. Maybe mammography works, but not very well. In any event, the effect, if it exists, is small enough that we just can't reliably detect it.

How good were the studies?

In the fall of 2001 a systematic review of all the mammography trials to date was completed by a group known as the Cochrane Collaboration, an international nonprofit organization that regularly reviews the evidence of health care interventions—a sort of *Consumer Reports* for medicine.[11] The article appeared in the *Lancet* and, soon after, on the front page of the *New York Times*.[12] Based on the rules of evidence that the Cochrane Collaboration uses for all interventions, many of the mammography trials were considered substandard—some not even worthy of inclusion in the review. This time the Canadian study stood out as one of the best-conducted studies, while the Swedish and American studies were identified as having the major flaws.

I have to admit, I was taken aback at the criticism of the American study. Maybe it was a bit of misplaced nationalism on my part. Maybe it was because the HIP was a "classic" study that I have always admired (it really was the first large-scale trial of cancer screening). Maybe it was because the findings of the HIP fit my beliefs about cancer testing: namely, that early detection—in this case mammography—works best when it is not too sensitive (that is, when the mammograms don't reveal every tiny abnormality of the breast).

So I wanted to critically examine what the Cochrane Collaboration had to say about the HIP study. Some of their complaints struck me as nitpicking. They were concerned, for example, that the number of patients in the mammography group was different in different publications (variously 30,131, 30,092, and 30,239), and likewise for the number of patients in the control group. While I find this kind of inconsistency irritating, I can't believe it has much effect on the study's findings. However, two problems were raised that definitely do call the validity of the study's findings into question—problems corroborated in the book written by the primary investigator of the HIP study.[13] I include them here to provide some flavor of the complex issues that arise in doing research on early cancer detection.

Problem 1: Questionable deaths were more likely to be called breast cancer deaths in the control group. The primary outcome of any breast cancer screening study is breast cancer death. While it is obvious that some women with breast cancer die from breast cancer, for others the cause of death is questionable. In the HIP study, 71 deaths were judged questionable in the breast exam/mammography group, versus 73 in the control group. That is about what one would expect: deaths were more or less equally likely to be considered questionable in the two groups. A committee then reviewed the deaths and decided that 13 questionable deaths in the mammography group were due to breast cancer, compared with 35 in the control group. That's not what one would expect: an extra 22 breast cancer deaths were assigned to the control group. For perspective, the total number of breast cancer deaths was 147 in the mammography group and 192 in the control group. In other words, the difference observed in the entire study was 45 breast cancer deaths. If the swing of 22 deaths in the death review process represented bias, then almost half of the observed effect of breast exam/mammography may not really exist.

Problem 2: Women with a prior history of breast cancer were less likely to be excluded from the control group. Ideally, women who have already had breast cancer would never be enrolled in a study of breast cancer screening (since screening is for people who have never had the cancer being tested for). But the HIP didn't evaluate women as they entered the study; instead it simply randomized women from the health plan's patient list. The result was that a number of women with a prior history of breast cancer were enrolled. Investigators later tried to exclude these women. Although one would expect that the mammography and the control group would contain about the same number of these women, somewhere between 400 and 500 (once again, the numbers are not consistent from publication to publication) more women were excluded for a prior history of breast cancer from the mammography group than from the control group.

How did that happen? There was systematic data collection on women receiving intervention. Thus, women with prior breast cancer were quickly identified and excluded from the group. But the control group did not receive such close attention (remember, these women did not even know they were in a study), and as a result women with prior breast cancer were less likely to be identified and excluded.

The problem is that women with a prior history of breast cancer are most likely to die from breast cancer. Although the investigators tried to remove these women when they reviewed deaths, that is hard to do reliably. Hence, the Cochrane Collaboration concluded that because the difference observed in the HIP study—45 more breast cancer deaths in the control group than in the intervention group—could be explained merely by the imbalance of women with prior breast cancer (whereas a balanced study might well have shown that mammography combined with clinical breast exam had no effect), the study should be excluded from their systematic review.

The reviewers raised similar concerns with three of the four Swedish trials, concerns that were subsequently contested by the investigators concerned.[14] Edinburgh was thrown out for the reasons alluded to earlier. Of the eight studies reviewed, therefore, only three even achieved the rating "medium quality": Malmö and the two Canadian trials. The issues raised by the Cochrane Collaboration highlight how difficult it is to run a good randomized trial of screening. Based on their analysis, the authors argued that "screening for breast cancer with mammography is unjustified."[15]

The general response of the medical and public health community to the Cochrane report was to dismiss the concerns and reaffirm previously held positions. The National Cancer Institute, U.S. Preventive Services Task Force, and American Cancer Society reiterated their view that there was sufficient evidence of the effectiveness of regular mammography. The World Health Organization issued a similar statement. Only an obscure group of experts from leading American medical institutions and government agencies had a different view. The PDQ Screening and Prevention Editorial Board, charged by the National Cancer Institute to produce data summaries for doctors and patients, concluded that they could not be sure about the true effect of mammography.

Learning the truth

What do I think the "truth" is about screening mammography? The truth is surely complex: whether or not mammography helps depends on a number of factors.

First, whether or not mammography helps depends on what it is being compared to. It is certainly better than nothing—when "nothing" is no mammography, no clinical breast exam, and low awareness of breast cancer in general. In fact, one of the side effects of promoting mammography may have been to increase women's awareness of breast cancer in general, such that they seek medical care more quickly when they find a breast lump in the course of normal life.

It is equally possible, however, that mammography is no better than a good clinical breast exam—though to be sure, it may be hard to get such an exam. The clinical breast exam done in the Canadian trial was carefully standardized, lengthy (5–15 minutes per patient), and generally performed by specially trained nurses. One of the advantages of mammography may be that it is easier to standardize the practice of the less than 10,000 American radiologists who read mammograms than it is to standardize the practice of the quarter of a million clinicians who might offer women clinical breast exams.[16] Nevertheless, the Canadian experience contains an important lesson: there is no obvious value to finding breast cancers that are so small they cannot be felt, such as most DCIS.[17]

It is also quite possible that routine screening mammography has nothing to offer women who are already sensitized to seek medical care when they find a breast lump in the course of normal life.[18] These women may have just the right amount of early detection.

Second, whether or not mammography helps depends on how one defines "helps." The truth is that mammography, like any screening test, has a mixture of outcomes. A few women probably have their lives extended—those who might have ignored a new lump or those who happen to have a mammogram at just the right time to catch and treat a fast-growing cancer. However, many women suffer the short-term anxiety of a cancer scare because of a falsely positive exam. Some women will know about a breast cancer earlier yet not have their death postponed; they simply live longer knowing they have breast cancer. Others will be diagnosed with pseudodisease and receive surgery and radiation unnecessarily. A few will even have their lives shortened by treatment.

To date, researchers have focused largely on the number of breast cancer deaths. Little attention has been given to measuring the adverse effects of breast cancer screening and treatment.

Finally, whether or not mammography helps depends on how it is done. Although we often use the word *mammography* as if it were a simple procedure, in reality it is a multistep process, each step having its own set of questions. How often should it be done? How many views should be taken? How much should the image be enhanced or magnified? How aggressively should the radiologist recommend biopsy for abnormalities? How aggressively should early abnormalities be treated? How these questions are answered will ultimately determine the effect of screening.

It is commonly assumed that more is always better: more frequent mammograms, more views, more magnification, more recommendations for biopsy, and more aggressive treatment will all lead to a better result. Of course, it is not that simple. It's possible, for example, that annual mammography for women in their 40s makes little difference, but doing it every three months would do some good, since younger women tend to have faster-growing cancers. Yet that might be too much radiation, as well as meaning more biopsies, more cancers found, and more people being treated.

What if instead of more we did less—might that not lead to a better result? To avoid a lot of pseudodisease and false positives, what if radiologists just looked for masses? The tiny microcalcifications associated with DCIS could be watchfully monitored (or ignored), but treatment could be deferred until it was clear that the abnormality was something to act on. As for treatment, might not some mammographically detected cancers be best treated not by surgery, but with hormonal manipulation (i.e., by stopping estrogen in those women who are on it and/or giving an antiestrogen like Tamoxifen)?[19] But then again, maybe if we do less, some cancers would be missed or undertreated. To understand these variables better, more research is needed.

Have you been paying attention? I just walked you through eight big studies that have been conducted over the past 40 years: almost half a million women entered in randomized trials of mammography; millions of dollars' worth of research. No cancer test has been more carefully studied. And we still need more research? The truth is, we do. There are other questions we need answers to before we can say how best to screen for breast cancer.

THE REAL CONSTRAINTS IN TESTING TESTS

Welcome to the real world of cancer detection research. Here are the hard facts. There are a lot of potential questions to ask. Studies can only take on one, maybe two questions at a time. They have to be big—because it takes lots of healthy people being tested to find a few cancers and, in turn, make a difference in preventing an even fewer number of cancer deaths. And the studies have important details to attend to—like how to determine why people died, and then deciding if that is all that matters.

Many options

Testing a cancer screening test actually involves studying the combined effect of early detection and early treatment. From the individual's perspective the question is, "Is a strategy of looking for and treating cancers before they become noticeable better than simply treating cancers at the point they become noticeable?" This question implies that two conditions must be met for screening to work: (1) the test must find cancers that will ultimately warrant treatment (i.e., not pseudodisease) and (2) treatment at the time of detection must be more effective than treatment at the time symptoms appear.

One of my closest colleagues makes the analogy that an early detection strategy is like a machine with lots of dials. Each dial has multiple possible settings: there's a dial to set the age to start screening, there's another for when to stop. There's a dial for how often to screen. There's a set of dials for technical controls (e.g., how many views? at what magnification?). Another set specifies how to interpret the test (e.g., what constitutes abnormal? when should a test be repeated? when should a different test be ordered?). Finally, there's a set of dials for treatment.

You can probably already guess that the "right" position for these dials is not up to the max. If you set the starting age dial too young, mostly what you do is worry a lot of young people with no possible benefit. If you set the stopping age too old, mostly what you do is detect a lot of pseudodisease and do a lot of unnecessary treatment in the elderly. If you test too frequently, you drive people—including doctors—crazy. If you make the test too sensitive, you get a lot of noise: false positives and pseudodisease. And if you treat too aggressively, the treatment becomes worse than the disease. If you turn all the dials up to the max, every person becomes a patient—some literally, all emotionally. You end up doing more harm than good.

So the "right" position is somewhere in the middle—just like setting brightness, hue, color, and contrast on your TV. The difference is that your TV gives instant feedback on your settings. You can quickly fine-tune the settings to improve the picture. Finding the right settings for a screening test, in contrast, takes time, money, and lots of volunteers.

Many people

How many healthy people need to be entered into a randomized trial to find out whether an early detection strategy (with a particular set of settings) reduces death? The short answer is, a lot. The longer answer is, it depends. It basically depends on two things: how likely a cancer death is and how much of a difference you want to detect.

To get a feel for this, let's start with a relatively easy case (from the researchers' perspective): screening cigarette smokers for lung cancer. It is an easy case because death is common, and when death is common it is easier to figure out whether intervention reduces the chance of death. Cigarette smokers face a relatively high risk of cancer death: among 1,000 middle-aged smokers, about 40 will die of lung cancer in the next 10 years. If you wanted to see whether lung cancer screening—early detection and early treatment—can cut that death rate in half (that is, from 40 to 20 per 1,000), the statisticians would tell you that you need to enroll 3,200 smokers in your study.[20]

Now, cutting a death rate in half is no walk in the park. It's more like climbing K2. No cancer test has ever achieved such a feat. But if you want to make sure you'll be able to detect a smaller effect, you need to study even more people. And the number needed rises exponentially. To see a 25 percent reduction in lung cancer deaths (from 40 to 30 per 1,000), for example, requires over 14,000 subjects; to see a 10 percent reduction in lung cancer deaths (from 40 to 36 per 1,000) requires almost 100,000.[21]

What if we move to a common cancer that affects smokers and non-smokers alike? Take colon cancer: among 1,000 middle-aged men and women, about 5 will die of colon cancer in the next 10 years. Now assume you want to know whether screening using, say, virtual colonoscopy is effective. A study designed to detect a 50 percent reduction in colon cancer mortality requires studying 25,000 people; detection of a 25 percent reduction requires studying 120,000 people; and a 10 percent reduction, 800,000 people. The numbers are a bit lower for breast cancer and quite a bit higher for the rarer cancers, such as ovarian cancer, pancreatic cancer, and lung cancer in nonsmokers.

Much ambiguity (why do people die?)

There's one more wrinkle I need to throw in here. These calculations were based on the assumption that researchers are trying to detect changes in the number of deaths due to a specific cancer. That's fine, so long as you are confident that the testing and early treatment process never leads anyone to die from something else. But I'm not especially confident of that. A woman who has part of her lung removed after an early lung cancer is found may be "cured" of cancer but die of pneumonia six months later. The surgery made pneumonia more likely, but it won't be counted as a lung cancer death. Similarly, a man who has part of his colon removed after a colon cancer is found may be "cured" of cancer but die of intestinal obstruction six months later. The surgery made the obstruction more likely, but it won't get counted as a colon cancer death. Other treatments for cancer may slightly increase the long-term chance of death from a secondary cause—for example, radiation seems to encourage heart disease, while chemotherapy may stimulate second cancers[22]—yet these deaths are not counted as deaths from the target cancer either. The problem is real: researchers reported that the number of deaths in cancer patients *due to something other than cancer* was 37 percent higher than in men and women of similar age.[23] Because these excess noncancer deaths occurred shortly after diagnosis, they concluded that a large proportion of them were due to cancer treatments.

And then there are all the people who don't have cancer but are nonetheless affected by the screening process. Some of the radiological studies and all the biopsies done as part of screening have risks. Sometimes doctors stumble onto other things along the way and start treatments they wouldn't have otherwise. Any death during the screening process won't get counted as cancer death, because these patients never had cancer in the first place.

Sure, such negative consequences are rare. But so are the benefits. Let me provide some context. The randomized trial showing the largest benefit of breast cancer screening, for example, found a difference of 22 breast cancer deaths (22 fewer among women screened than among those not screened) among a total of 1,000 deaths overall; the trial showing the largest benefit of colon cancer screening found a difference of 40 colon cancer deaths among a total of 6,000 deaths overall.[24] All it would take is a few deaths somehow related to screening and the positive effects would diminish, or even disappear.

Before we set about persuading healthy people to go looking for cancer, I think we owe it to them to be damn sure that cancer detection in fact lowers overall death rates. I don't want to worry about how somebody somewhere decided why someone died.[25] I don't want to worry that we are trading off one cause of death for another. And I believe a lower chance of death is what most people expect we mean when we say things like "screening works" or "screening can save lives."

But to be sure we are lowering overall death rates means we have to study even more people. As you saw above, to detect a 25 percent reduction in colon cancer deaths requires studying 120,000 people. But colon cancer represents at most 4 percent of all deaths. Looking for a 25 percent reduction in deaths from a disease that is responsible for 4 percent of all deaths means we'd like to reliably detect a 1 percent drop in total death rate (25 percent × 4 percent). The price for this power? A study involving over a million people . . .[26]

Many researchers involved in early cancer detection say simply, "It can't be done"; "It's just too big." What they are really saying is, "We can't be sure whether a strategy of early cancer detection truly saves lives." I don't know what the right answer is, but I think we have one of two choices: either do the study or publicly acknowledge that we cannot be sure whether early detection lengthens, shortens, or has no effect on how long people live. And we should be clear that if it takes so many people to find out for sure, then the benefit must be, at best, small.

Much complexity (is living all that matters?)

Let's say that, conceptually at least, we had a really big, well-performed study that definitively answered the question "Does this particular early detection strategy allow people to live longer?" Even if the answer was unambiguously yes (or no), most of us would probably want to know about other effects. The testing strategy may diminish suffering for those otherwise destined to develop advanced cancer (by finding and treating cancer early, pain and disability may be reduced). But testing is also likely to increase the suffering of others: those who don't have cancer and those who have pseudodisease (by increasing the number of people who undergo extensive evaluation and are treated). There is undoubtedly some psychological morbidity as well, not only from unnecessary cancer scares, but also from the "you might have cancer" fear that must be promulgated to persuade healthy people to get tested in the first place.

In the final analysis, the net effect of screening requires a rather substantial equation:

| Years of life saved by early treatment | + | Morbidity avoided by early treatment | + | Worry caused by promoting fear about hidden cancers | + | Anguish from cancer "scares" | + | Morbidity from unnecessary treatment | + | Years of life lost from treatment | = | Net effect of test |

Quite honestly, most of us would be comfortable ignoring all those inter-mediate terms if the years of life benefit was really big. But as I explained in Chapter 1, most of the time it isn't. So those other terms become im-portant. And that raises thorny measurement issues. While you can count the number of additional mastectomies done following a strategy of mammography screening, for example, how do you measure morbidity from the operation? And if you think that's tough, what about measuring the extent to which the promotion of mammography leads to general fear about breast cancer?

Some researchers are at work trying to measure these hard-to-quantify outcomes. But even if they develop appropriate measurement tools, poli-cymakers are left with a more basic problem: the numbers never add up. How do you balance an unnecessary mastectomy in woman A against 10 years' more life for woman B? What do you think? Would you say 10 un-necessary mastectomies equal 10 years of life? I think different people would say different things. Obviously there is no right answer—and that is the point. The most we can expect from research is some feel for how big each of the terms in the equation is. Individuals will need to decide for them-selves which numbers matter and how to put them together.

GENETIC TESTING

It is difficult to talk about medical research these days without saying something about genes. There is a tremendous amount of enthusiasm out there for genetic testing and gene therapy. Some of this is perfectly un-derstandable: fantastic things *are* being learned. But there is also a fair amount of irrational exuberance, and maybe even a little self-promotion. Given the hoopla, a casual observer could be forgiven for thinking that knowledge about the human genome has put us on the verge of winning the war on cancer. The reality is, it has been a war we have been on the verge of winning for some 30 years. We have made progress, but progress comes slowly. Genetic researchers would do well to be a bit more circum-spect about what people can and cannot expect.

Since this is a book about cancer testing, I will confine my comments to genetic testing and avoid gene therapy. First, though, let me define my terms. *Genetic testing* really involves the search for various molecules—not just genes per se, but also the molecules that the genes code for (called gene products). And there are really two very different settings for such molecular testing: testing healthy people to better characterize their risk of cancer, on the one hand, and testing people who already have cancer to better characterize the cancer, on the other.

Testing people for cancer risk

One vision of the future is that all young adults, say at age 20, would undergo genetic testing to learn about their risk for major diseases such as heart disease, psychiatric disorders, diabetes, and cancer. It is a vision articulated by the head of the Human Genome Project, Francis Collins, who in a report to Congress stated that "a baseline genome scan could give patients and health care providers helpful information about an individual's disease risk profile and point to which prevention strategies—when available—should be put into place."[27] While I have no doubt that a genome scan could provide such information, I'm a little less sanguine about the "helpful" part. Let me tell you two reasons why.

Genetic tests can't erase the uncertainty of who will get cancer. Doctors didn't need to be able to read DNA to know that some cancers have a strong genetic component. It's obvious: there are families in which many members develop the same cancer at a relatively young age. It is for people in these families that genetic tests are arguably the most useful. A positive test means you have the cancer gene, a negative test means you don't.[28] But a positive test doesn't mean you definitely will get cancer, and, more important, a negative test doesn't mean you won't.

Take the most familiar genetic test, for BRCA1, the abnormal gene associated with breast cancer. Consider a 30-year-old female. If she has a positive test, her risk of developing breast cancer by age 70 is around 50 percent.[29] (That is simply the chance of being diagnosed with cancer, not the chance of dying from it.) If she has a negative test, her risk of the same is just a little below average—around 10 percent. That's because most breast cancers—like most other cancers—are not the result of a single genetic defect.

This information may be helpful to some and not others. Whether it is helpful hinges on how the result affects the course of action: how mammography is used, whether the woman decides to undergo immediate mastectomy, whether she changes how she lives her life. The test is also helpful if the individual tested is certain she will take one course of action facing a probability of 50 percent and a different one facing a probability of 10 percent. But if she is going to do the same thing either way, then I'd argue the test isn't really helpful. Certainly, it would be even more helpful if it better distinguished the probabilities: if positive meant 100 percent chance and negative meant no chance. But that isn't the case.

Most of us don't have such a strong family history for cancer. And most of the cancers treated by doctors don't have strong single-gene origins. Instead, most cancers are the result of multiple genetic alterations in an organism being exposed to multiple environmental factors (some of which occur naturally). And even if we could catalog every possible genetic alteration (which is conceivable) and all the environmental influences at play (a tougher nut to crack), we can never be certain about the role of chance. That's right: some people get cancer simply because of bad luck.

So what can most of us expect from genetic testing? By testing multiple genes, we will be better able to estimate an individual's risk of developing certain cancers. Of course, we have been able to provide a crude estimate of risk, based on age, race, and sex, for many years. A genome scan will merely further refine this risk. But for most of us the risk refinements will probably fall within a fairly narrow range of relatively low probabilities: lowering it from 10 to 5 percent, or raising it from 2 to 6 percent.[30] Although some may emphasize that we've been able to inform people that their risk is "cut in half" or "increased threefold," I doubt that will provide a strong enough rationale for a change in behavior.

Genetic tests can't answer the question of what to do next. Imagine you are a 20-year-old female having just undergone a baseline genome scan. Your risk profile shows you have an 8.5 percent chance of developing ovarian cancer sometime in your life. That's four times the risk for an "average" woman. You don't have the aberration strongly associated with an increased risk of lung cancer in both smokers and nonsmokers, meaning your risk for this cancer is well below average. You also have a DNA variant that some researchers believe increases your risk of breast cancer by almost 50 percent, although your doctor reassures you that this point has seen considerable debate in the literature recently. Another gene variant is present that substantially increases your risk for a rare form of a salivary gland cancer, but it's so rare that your doctor suggests you forget about it. Otherwise your risk for the other common cancers is about average.

Your genome scan also provides information about other diseases. Your risk of heart disease is 25 percent higher than normal—and your doctor reminds you that you need to take that seriously, since heart disease is by far the major cause of death across the span of life. This finding doesn't really surprise you because your mother had a heart attack a couple of years ago. The same aberration that lowers your risk of lung cancer seems to also lower your risk of death from pneumonia or influenza (although this won't be important until you are much older). Finally, you have a form of a gene that has been found to increase the risk of stroke, but lowers the risk of blindness. Researchers are actively working to better quantify this relationship.

Now what? Oops, the genome doesn't answer that question. Some might argue that the first step would be to deal with the fourfold increase in the risk of ovarian cancer—perhaps by removing your ovaries. Others might point out that heart disease is a more likely cause of death for you—particularly after age 50. Taking out the ovaries and thus inducing menopause might only increase your risk. Another person might suggest removing your ovaries and starting estrogen replacement, which might shield against heart disease—though someone else would no doubt point out that that will increase your risk of breast cancer.

Issues bigger than medical care arise as well. What if you want to have children? Maybe you should start now rather than waiting. But what if you are unmarried and were planning to stay that way for at least another five years? Well, perhaps you should adjust your vision of the future. Then again, maybe you shouldn't.

Perhaps I am guilty of creating a scenario where the choices are too stark. There is, of course, a middle ground: the best thing might be to have regular (say annual) abdominal ultrasounds. But even this approach is not innocuous. As we have seen, ultrasounds can identify many abnormalities on the kidney. And radiologists can't always distinguish between benign ovarian cysts and ovarian cancer. A strategy of annual abdominal ultrasounds beginning in women 20 years of age is bound to lead to frequent biopsies and, occasionally, unnecessary removal of ovaries and kidneys.

To know whether the regular ultrasound strategy helped more than it hurt would require a randomized trial. But that would be very difficult for two reasons. First, it would need to be restricted to a select group of women: those with the gene associated with ovarian cancer. Second, it would need to follow them for a very long time: from their 20s into their 40s and 50s. And the same sort of research would be needed for each gene abnormality–early detection strategy combination.

But aren't we obligated to make such an effort before we embark on this kind of genetic testing? Otherwise, all we are doing is getting young people to focus prematurely on death (and perhaps distracting them from their highest risk for death in the near term: accidents). If we really have little idea of what to do differently, this kind of broad-based genetic testing merely adds clutter. Moreover, it further distracts from the practice of medicine: rather than making sick people well, we end up making well people sick.

Testing cancers for prognosis

I am more optimistic about what genetic testing might mean for patients who have already been diagnosed with cancer. The more we learn about the genes that control cancer cell growth, the better able we will be to predict which cancers will grow fast and which will not. We'll also be better placed to distinguish pseudodisease from aggressive cancer. And we'll be better able to predict the host response and tailor therapy to the specific disease.

Recently, for example, researchers examined some 5,000 genes in each of 78 early breast cancer cases.[31] Because these specimens had been collected years earlier, the researchers knew which breast cancers ultimately went on to produce distant metastases (that is, which ones were aggressive). They found that a molecular profile of 70 genes could accurately predict which cancers were aggressive and which were not. When they tested their approach on a new set of 19 cancers, moreover, it worked very well.

This is a tremendous step forward. I don't want to downplay the importance of findings such as these. Genetic testing of early cancer *will* help us predict which cancers need aggressive treatment, which ones need standard treatment, and which ones can be watched.

But it will never be perfect. Tumor markers and genes can provide probabilities, but not definitive answers. Consider the research I just described. If the molecular profile diagnosed a cancer as aggressive, 70 percent of the time it was right—but 30 percent of the time it was wrong. And if the profile diagnosed a cancer as *not* aggressive, 90 percent of the time it was right—and 10 percent of the time wrong. Even with the most complete information, the "right answer" may not be obvious. "You have a .5 cm growth that, based on its gene expression profile, has less than a 10 percent chance of metastasizing in the next five years." That's important information. But now what should you do?

RESEARCH THAT REALLY NEEDS TO BE DONE

Maybe we are thinking about cancer the wrong way. Medicine's approach to date has focused on finding cancer as early as possible and acting as quickly as possible. But you now know there's a price for getting too far ahead of the game: the price of unnecessary worry, unnecessary treatment, finding too much cancer, disagreement about who has cancer, and distraction from more pressing concerns.

Cancer is a dynamic process in which many things must go wrong. It can be imagined as a cascade of events, in which a number of opportunities exist to stop the process (Figure 17). The process starts when a cell experiences some genetic damage: a DNA mutation. In fact, this kind of damage is believed to be a very common occurrence. The vast majority of the time, the mutation is repaired—but sometimes it's not. Then if there is a second mutation and another repair failure, the cell may become irrevo-

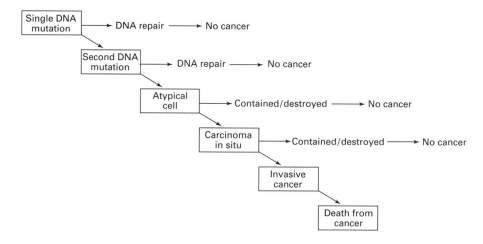

Figure 17.   Cancer as a multistep process that need not necessarily progress.

cably damaged. Most of the time these atypical cells self-destruct or are recognized by the body's defense system—but sometimes they start to replicate and go unchecked. As collections of abnormal cells form, the host's immune response is usually activated—but again, sometimes it's not. So while we all have DNA mutations, only a few of us die from cancer. One step does not necessarily lead to another.

Yet we often act as if it does. Our current approach to cancer diagnosis and intervention seems to assume that the process proceeds in lockstep. Pathologists are asked to make a judgment based on a few cells, a judgment that may initiate a chain of aggressive reactions. But the pathologist is trying to predict the occurrence of a dynamic process (spreading throughout the body, ending in death) based on a static observation (the appearance of cells under the microscope) early in the process. What we really need to learn more about is the dynamics of early cancer.

Some of the genetic testing of the cancers themselves can help move us in this direction. But the use of genetic testing also calls for a heretical approach: waiting and simply watching. We know that some abnormalities that meet the cellular definition of cancer won't progress and that some small abnormalities on a scan today may not be there tomorrow. The best way to sort these cases out may be to do research on a more dynamic diagnostic process—one that involves repeated measurements over time.

SUMMARY

It is very difficult to know whether our interventions to detect early forms of cancers really help people. A well-designed study of a cancer screening test takes many years, requires millions of dollars, and involves thousands of volunteers. More studies really are needed. To do them we will need people like you to participate. We need studies that measure the full range of positive and negative events that can occur following testing. And we need to carefully consider one outcome about which there is no debate, an outcome that all patients care about: death, no matter what the cause.

But no one should expect that we will learn everything. There will always be more questions than we can answer. Genetic testing may help answer some of these, but it will raise many more. These tests will never be definitive; they can't tell you that you definitely will or will not get cancer. Instead, genetic tests only identify who is at higher and lower risk— in turn raising more questions about when, whether, and how to look for cancer. If we want to test for cancer, whether by using biochemical tests, imaging studies, or genetic profiles, we must accept that there will always be a fair amount of guesswork about the right thing to do once a positive result is arrived at.

Our approach to testing must reflect the fact that cancer is a complex dynamic process. If we are going to look for early cancer, we may need to study a new diagnostic strategy: watchful waiting. It is entirely possible that we would do better with a little bit more watching and a little less action.

TEN *Develop a strategy that works for you*

"Chances are you're fine. But why take chances?"

"Take the test, not the chance."

"Early warning signs of colon cancer: You feel great. You have a healthy appetite. You're only 50."

"Mammograms: The chance of a lifetime."

Every day you can see strong messages in the media encouraging you to get tested for cancer. And you can be sure there will be no let-up in the near future. Some will try to scare you into action. Others will appeal to your sense of reason. Most will imply that doctors are sure that early cancer detection is always the best strategy. Few, if any, will communicate any reason you would not want to be tested. Their theme will be consistent: the benefits of testing are certain, the downsides nonexistent—or at most, trivial.

Having read this book, you now know that the reality of cancer testing is quite the reverse. It is the downsides that are certain, while the benefits—in most cases—are unclear. Even so, I am not suggesting that testing healthy people for cancer is never helpful. The possibility that you might benefit from screening means that you face a genuine, and difficult, decision.

In this chapter I will try to help you think through that decision. Frankly, this was the most difficult chapter for me to write. Those of us engaged in research are much more comfortable dealing with questions about what is going on—the kinds of questions I have addressed so far in this book. We are less comfortable with the logical follow-up question: "What should I do?" Let's try to think about that together.

SCARED TO DEATH

Soon after I started writing this book I was asked to give a talk explaining some of the downsides of cancer testing. The talk, sponsored by the Dartmouth Community Medical School, was part of a larger effort to expose the general public to recent scientific developments in medicine and to encourage participation in current medical debates. Over a hundred people came; most were of an age for which cancer screening is directly relevant. The group was very engaged and, judging by their questions, understood well the problems I was posing.

Nonetheless, many of the ideas I presented were clearly disturbing to this audience. People were surprised at how few cancer tests had been studied rigorously and, in those that had, how little effect screening had on the number of deaths in general (Chapter 1). While the notion of false positive results and cascades of testing were familiar (Chapter 2), the idea that people might be treated unnecessarily or have a cancer found that they would rather not know about was not (Chapters 3 and 4). But most disconcerting was the general uncertainty about who really had cancer— particularly the idea that different pathologists might say different things (Chapter 5).

One woman was particularly frustrated. She pointed out that I had presented a lot of problems without providing an obvious course of action. I think she understood that there were no simple answers and found that frightening. She said, "At some point don't we have to decide how much faith we have in our general internist, our radiologist, and our pathologist? We can't go through life wondering what else is lingering beneath the surface. I fear as you tell people to be advocates for their own health care, you run the risk of scaring them to death."

I agree. The current tendency is to expect people to take more responsibility for their health and to participate more actively in medical decision making. One of the reasons I wrote this book is that I support this approach. But as in all things, moderation is called for. People cannot assume sole responsibility for their own health; much illness is outside personal control (so let's not blame people for being sick). And doctors should not assign sole responsibility for decision making to the patient. We have to be careful not to be heard as saying, "I don't care what you do, it's your decision." Most patients look to their doctor for guidance while they actively participate in medical decision making. Some want doctors to make decisions for them, and that's okay too. If being an "advocate for your own health care" translates into making decisions without any input from your doctor, it is easy to understand how people can become "scared to death." No one wants to make important medical decisions alone.

But the woman's statement contains another idea, an insight into how people get scared to death in the first place: they worry about what *might* be going on. By now you probably understand that this is one of my fundamental concerns about the whole enterprise of testing for cancer: it causes people to worry about what might be going wrong inside them. How you feel about this kind of "dis-ease" being spread by the medical system is a good place to start in addressing the question "What should I do?"

ASK YOURSELF WHAT YOU WANT FROM MEDICAL CARE

As I said in the introduction, the dominant cancer prevention strategy in American medicine today is to look for cancer in people who have no symptoms. Given the problems discussed in this book, you will want to gauge your own reaction to this approach. How we perceive health is a choice: you may assume you are healthy until proven otherwise or assume that a problem may exist until proven otherwise. How much effort, emotional and otherwise, do you want to devote to looking for things wrong when you feel well? To what extent would you rather focus on *being* well when you feel well?

Many forces combine to make medical care a more prominent part of all of our lives—even when we are well. Scientific advances mean more is possible; increased societal affluence means more is affordable. And size of the market—lots of healthy people—means there are strong economic incentives to promote preventive services for the well. But it is important to think about how working to avoid death might affect your experience of life. Do you see medical care as a way to deal with problems you observe, or as a vehicle to find those problems you are not aware of? Another way to phrase the question might be: Do you want to focus your efforts on staying well or on avoiding death? Of course, there are more than two choices; our relationship to medical care falls along a spectrum:

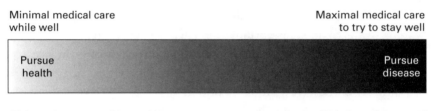

Minimal medical care while well	Maximal medical care to try to stay well
Pursue health	Pursue disease

Risk: perhaps a small increase in chance of cancer death *Risk: larger chance of medicalization and overtreatment*

You might find it useful to think about where you are on it.

You also need to think about how you feel about cancer in particular. A few questions may help you initiate the process. Do you have a particular interest in avoiding dying from cancer? Would you gladly trade a cancer death for any other? Would you, perhaps, do everything you can to avoid it—even at the price of a greater likelihood that you will be diagnosed with cancer and suffer harms from treatment? Feelings like this argue for testing: desiring at all costs to avoid death, people who feel this way are quite willing to allow medical care a large role in their life.

Others, however, may prefer to focus on being healthy (rather than trying to procure health) and choose to minimize medical contact while they feel well. They may deliberately trade off a small increase in the risk of cancer death for the very real benefits of avoiding medicalization, excessive diagnosis, and overtreatment. People who feel this way prefer to work to stay well, reserving medical care for problems as they present themselves.

Pursuing disease is not at all the same as pursuing health. In fact, they easily conflict. It can be quite difficult to promote wellness when you are actively looking for things to be wrong.

Of course, different people feel differently about cancer. And different people have different approaches to life. So we should expect that people will make different decisions about testing.

ASK YOUR DOCTOR THREE SIMPLE QUESTIONS

Answering the question "What should I do?" may involve a conversation with your doctor. Before having that conversation, however, take a minute to put yourself in his or her shoes. Think about the question of testing from your doctor's standpoint.

Doctors can hardly go wrong suggesting a test. If the test is normal, we can offer patients the reassurance that they are well. If the test is abnormal but the patient is subsequently shown not to have cancer, the patient is so relieved that questions about the original decision to test are unlikely to be raised. And if the patient is found to have cancer, there is the silver lining: we caught it early. The question of whether the test or the diagnosis was necessary will never be raised.

But doctors can go wrong if we fail to order a test—especially if another doctor recommends it later, in which case our patients may feel that we were somehow derelict in our duties. If our patient then develops and dies from an advanced cancer, we will be the one who missed it. Few will consider that the cancer might not have been present earlier or, if present, that it might not have been any more treatable.

Asking questions will help move your doctor beyond this kind of calculus. I know that some patients hesitate to ask their doctor questions. However, asking questions is the only way to participate in the decision. And you may be pleasantly surprised by your doctor's reaction. (I, for one, am always a little nervous when a patient agrees to a course of action without asking any questions.) Here are the three questions I suggest that you focus on when the issue of testing is raised.

Why are you suggesting the test? This is a good question to start the conversation. The answer should give you some insight into how carefully your practitioner has thought about the test and how strongly she believes in it. I'm not suggesting that beliefs should be the deciding factor, but it is a reasonable place to start. If applicable—depending on age and gender— you might ask whether the doctor undergoes this test herself, or whether she recommends it for her parents.

You may learn from this exchange that your practitioner is dogmatic, which suggests that you will not get far with further questions. Or you may learn that she has thought a great deal about the issue and has some reservations about testing. Perhaps the test is "recommended" or there is some institutional goal to be met (it is always fair to ask, "Are you under any pressure to test?"). Simply by asking the question "Why test?" you indicate that you know there are two sides to the testing issue. At the same time, you make clear to your provider that you are open to the idea of not being tested.

Has there been a randomized trial of screening for this cancer? This is a tougher question, one to which your doctor may not know the answer. If he does, however, the answer will quite possibly be no. But in some cases the answer will be yes, and then a follow-up question is called for: *What did it show?*

This question will help you determine whether the test has been found to have any real benefits.[1] If so, you may also get a feel for how much benefit there is. Don't expect to learn about the harms of testing from this question—just know they are always there. By now it will be obvious to your doctor that you want to make a considered decision.

What will we do if my test is positive? This is a pretty basic question, but it is not asked often enough. It helps you learn about the next step before you take the first. If for whatever reason you would choose not to take that next step, it makes no sense for you to be tested; a positive result will only give you information you will not use, and it will almost certainly make you worry.

This question tells your doctor that you are thinking ahead. You are aware that a positive test may trigger a cascade of subsequent events, and you'd like to have some sense of what these events might be and, if possible, how likely they are.

CONSIDER WHO YOU ARE

The decision to be tested for cancer can be looked on as a gamble. While most people are unaffected by testing, a few will be helped, and some will be hurt. To be helped you must have a cancer you are destined to die from if not tested. Note that that sentence contains two requirements: (1) the cancer must be one that is destined to be lethal and (2) it must be treatable if found by the test but not treatable if found later.

It is a little harder to define who will be hurt. Two groups can be singled out: those who will die of cancer anyway—with or without testing; and those not destined to die of cancer (that is, those destined to die of something else). To be hurt, people from these groups must suffer a considerable loss attributable to the testing process: they may experience undue anxiety, or learn about their cancer years before it was destined to become a problem, or experience morbidity (and occasional mortality) from a treatment that wasn't needed.

So you might envision two strategies to improve the odds of "winning": increase the chances of being helped and decrease the chances of being hurt. In this gamble, we can identify groups of people who are more likely to come out on top:

People at high risk to die of the cancer being sought. If the combination of early detection and treatment works, it is most likely to work in high-risk people: those with strong family histories (genetic predisposition) or with substantial exposure to known carcinogens. Abnormal test results in these people are much more likely to be significant and much less likely to be false positives. These people are more likely than most to have real disease—not pseudodisease. In short, the more likely you are to get the cancer, the more likely the potential benefit from testing exceeds the potential harm, and the more reason there is to try to find cancer early.

People in relatively good health. Remember, the whole idea of early detection is to try to get ahead of the cancer. Getting ahead is measured in terms of years. For any of this effort to be worth it, you should have a reasonable expectation that you will be alive in the next decade.

The careful reader may note a contradiction between these two groups of people. Because the risk of dying of cancer rises with age, the defining characteristic of the first group argues for screening the old. Yet because life expectancy decreases with age, the second argues for screening the young. As with many things, the ideal is somewhere in the middle. Testing for cancer is most likely to benefit those who have both a considerable risk for cancer and a considerable life expectancy—that is, middle-aged people, roughly age 50 to 70.

People who can be patient. The most important cancers tend to announce themselves clearly: the tests are unambiguously abnormal and all observers agree that it is cancer. But you need to be ready for small, questionable abnormalities as well. Probably the best way to minimize the harmful effects of screening is to be willing to take some time with these. Too often, big decisions are made based on a single observation, when it makes better sense to wait and take further readings. The best response to an abnormal test, therefore, may be to check it again in a few months. When one pathologist says the abnormality is a small early cancer, it may be worthwhile to ask a second pathologist to take a look. And even when "cancer" is agreed on, it may make sense to wait and be sure the cancer is really growing.

Watchful waiting can be hard. Patience takes courage. Moreover, it seems contrary to the conventional wisdom about cancer, which is that one must act fast. But patience *is* often a virtue, and it can help protect you from overtreatment.

People whose doctors understand that early detection is a two-edged sword. To be honest, watchful waiting is hard for doctors too. Think about it: I'm watching a patient's cancer. While the semiannual scan has become rou-

tine for him, I feel like I am waiting to be proved wrong. I think I'm doing the right thing, but I'll never know for certain until he dies from something else. Had we made a decision to take the cancer out, I could never
be proved wrong—even if he died on the operating table. To avoid being
proved wrong, it is always safer for the doctor to treat—even if that is not
the best course for the patient.

This kind of patience does not come easily for doctors. Many of us are
from the "when in doubt, cut it out" school. Watching an early cancer en-
tails a considerable paradigm shift. Because it is no fun to fight your doctor on this issue, you will want to make sure your doctor is able to see
both sides. You want a doctor who can see beyond simply doing everything possible to avoid "missing cancer," who understands that acting on
every abnormality is *over*reacting—a prescription for overdiagnosis and
overtreatment.

PRUDENT POLICIES

So far I have suggested ways of gathering information that might be relevant to your decision. I have avoided being prescriptive—for ultimately,
the decision is your own. But there are four policies I do want to be more
directive about. I believe each can help minimize some of the problems
of testing.

Tell your doctor you understand there are reasons not to be tested. Doctors assume patients want tests. Consequently, our default action is generally to
order them—even when we think it may not be the most sensible thing
to do. You can change that dynamic, however: tell your doctor that you
understand there can be downsides to testing and that you would like to
pursue a more balanced approach. In other words, give your doctor permission to consider not testing. It may lead to a more considered style of
practice—not just with regard to testing, but with regard to medical care
in general.

Don't overreact to abnormal test results. If you are tested, you need to be
ready for a result that is abnormal, but not markedly so. The aggressive

approach is "to get to the bottom of things" with additional tests and/or biopsy. Some doctors pursue this strategy because they think it is the right one, but many pursue it because they think it is what patients want or because they fear being sued for malpractice. All abnormal tests are not equal, though, and while markedly abnormal results are often indicative of real disease, barely abnormal results are generally where false positive tests and pseudodisease come from. So this is where patience comes in: it generally makes more sense to repeat the test in a few months than to act now. You have a choice about what to do following abnormal Pap smears, suspicious mammograms, and slightly elevated PSAs. Many doctors recognize the prudent approach is to repeat the test at a later date. They will be pleasantly surprised if you have considered this option as well.

Have another pathologist evaluate small cancers. If you have a small cancer diagnosed or if there is any ambiguity about the diagnosis, consider having a second pathologist look at the tissue. But do your best to ensure the second reading is truly independent of the first—that is, that the second pathologist does not know the first diagnosis. This suggestion doesn't mean I think pathologists are a bunch of sheep, simply that they are human. As an analogy I like to quote an expert on underwater recovery operations, whose simple rule for the technicians viewing video imagery of objects in a shipwreck is that no one can say aloud what he thinks he sees; instead, each writes down his independent interpretation. Otherwise, they all arrive at a "conclusion that has more to do with social dynamics . . . than the reality of the situation."[2] Independent observations are every bit as important in pathology as in recovery operations. Try to find a second pathologist who doesn't work with—or better yet, doesn't even know—the first. Various websites exist that can help with getting a second opinion.[3]

Consider a menu of treatment options. Finally, there is the question of what to do about a cancer detected by screening. Do not get pushed to act before you have had time to think. Most people overestimate the importance of acting quickly; remember that the chance you caught a cancer that was destined to kill you during the one week you could prevent it from killing you is infinitesimally small. You have time to think through your decision, and you should take the time to learn about the disease and your treatment options—including the more conservative ones. You should also know that the screen-detected cancer is bound to be less aggressive than the cancer with symptoms. And if pathologists disagree about whether cancer is present in the first place, the growth is likely to be even less aggressive. These are the cases where simply watching the abnormality for a few months may be the best course of action.

WRONG REASONS TO BE TESTED

While there may be no wrong decisions, there are certainly wrong reasons to be tested. Two in particular stand out.

Someone else wants you to. One wrong reason to be tested is because you think it will please someone else. Spouses and other family members come to mind here; so do close friends. But another person some may feel obliged to please is the doctor. Patients may worry that they will disappoint their doctor and that a disappointed doctor might abandon them. For most primary care practitioners, this concern is unwarranted. Practitioners as a rule value highly the principle of patient autonomy; in other words, we respect what individual patients want. Although a few doctors may become angry with patients who do not do as they say, that is a bad reason to be tested for cancer—and probably a good reason to find another practitioner.

The powerful (and misleading) personal anecdote. You have heard the stories, whether from friends and acquaintances or propagated in the media. A person whose "life was saved by a test"; another who died simply because his cancer wasn't "caught early." That's powerful stuff. But while the facts of the individual cases may be accurate, the conclusion that cancer testing must save lives is not.

Stories are not a reason to get tested for cancer. People whose lives were allegedly saved may not have needed treatment, or they may have been treated just as successfully years later. Or they may die of their cancer anyway and simply end up having known about it longer. People whose lives were allegedly lost by the lack of testing may not have been treated any more successfully with early diagnosis, or testing may have missed the cancer. The reason to get tested for cancer is because it really saves lives (something that takes thousands of cases to prove), not because someone testifies that her own life was saved or that someone else's could have been.

MAINTAIN PERSPECTIVE

The most important thing to realize is that there is no one right way to answer the question of whether to be tested. Two doctors who have devoted most of their careers to medical decision making—one of whom also served as editor-in-chief of the *New England Journal of Medicine* for almost a decade—have referred to the close calls in screening as "toss-ups": "situations in which the consequences of different decisions are, on average, virtually identical."[4] They go on to argue that under these circumstances it is impossible to make a bad decision about what to do next. But they are also quick to add that it is important for doctors to identify clearly those situations that qualify as toss-ups so that patients can focus on more personal considerations.

These doctors are referring to what are arguably the most widely recognized close calls in screening: mammography for women in their 40s and PSA testing. But the notion of a toss-up applies to screening decisions in general.[5] And in every close call, your personal considerations matter.

On one side, there is the potential benefit of screening: a lower risk of death. But as you saw in the last chapter, this benefit is so rare that it is exceedingly difficult to determine whether it in fact exists—much less measure it.

On the other side are the potential harms—the subject of most of this book. They are more common than the benefits, but for the most part of less consequence. Or let me be more specific: the harms with arguably the least consequence—cancer scares and additional testing—are quite common, while those with the greatest consequence—complications and/or death from unnecessary treatment—are very uncommon.

For most people, however, the most likely outcome of cancer testing is nothing: neither benefit nor harm. So unless you seek out every cancer test ever developed and undergo them frequently (an approach where the risks are really too high), it is hard to go too wrong. But it is still important to think about the decision, because not every choice will necessarily be right for you.

SUMMARY

Making a decision about cancer testing, like most medical decisions, involves weighing potential benefits and harms. Most people believe that there are no harms to testing; my interest in writing this book is to help people understand that there are in fact two sides to the issue. Let me reiterate that this message applies to testing people who *do not* have symptoms; it does not apply to testing people who are sick. And I am not suggesting that screening is always the wrong thing to do. There are times to test and times not to test. I also want people to be prepared for the fact that there is not and never will be a definitive "answer" about screening, no matter how much research is done.

Deciding whether to be tested for cancer involves much more than knowing the facts. While evidence of benefit or harm is relevant to the decision, so too are your own situation and your own values. Take the time to consider them. Make a proactive choice. If you choose not to go looking for cancer, feel good about staying healthy and staying out of doctors' offices. If you choose to go looking for cancer, feel good about trying to find disease early and managing it prudently.

I want to return to the woman's question about having faith in one's doctor. My response is, yes, you should have faith in your doctor. But not the old-fashioned type of faith, the faith that he or she always has the right answer. Instead I see something much richer—and much more realistic.

You can trust that your doctor understands that the world of health care is highly complex, much more so than is generally portrayed in books, magazines, and the electronic media. You can trust that your doctor knows there is much uncertainty in medical care. And if your doctor recognizes that you appreciate the complexity and uncertainty as well, you should have faith that you can have a different kind of relationship with your doctor—one that produces better decisions on your behalf.

Summary of cancers
discussed in this book

	New cases	Deaths	Average years of life lost per death[1]	Cumulative years of life lost[2]	Rank[3]
Lung cancer[4]	171,900	157,200	15	2,287,000	1
Breast cancer	212,600	40,200	19	779,000	2
Colon cancer	147,500	57,100	13	767,000	3
Prostate cancer	220,900	28,900	10	275,000	8
Renal cell carcinoma (kidney cancer)	31,900	11,900	15	180,000	13
Melanoma[5]	54,200	7,600	18	138,000	15
Cervical cancer	12,200	4,100	26	106,000	19
Thyroid cancer	22,000	1,400	—	nr	—
Neuroblastoma	600	nr	—	nr	—

SOURCE: 2003 data release, Surveillance, Epidemiology, and End Results (SEER) Program, National Cancer Institute.

NOTE: nr = not reported.

[1] This column shows the number of years a typical patient would be expected to live if he or she did not die from the cancer (i.e., normal life expectancy minus the age of death). The numbers have been rounded.

[2] This measure is the product of two factors: (1) how many people died and (2) how many years they would be expected to live if they did not have cancer. Although not as familiar as the number of deaths, this is the best measure of the true burden of death from cancer.

[3] This ranking is based on the cumulative number of years of life lost from all cancer deaths reported in the United States in 2003.

[4] If there were no cigarette smoking in the United States, the numbers in this row would be one-tenth as big.

[5] Melanoma is the deadliest form of skin cancer. Other forms (e.g., basal cell, squamous cell) are much more common but rarely, if ever, cause death.

GLOSSARY

absolute risk

The actual chance of experiencing a particular event in a defined time period. In cancer, absolute risk is typically expressed per 1,000 or per 100,000. For a person age 50, for example, the absolute risk of death from colon cancer in the next 10 years is 3 per 1,000. *See also* relative risk.

barium enema

A test in which a tube is inserted in the rectum and a thick fluid is allowed to flow up the colon by gravity. Because the fluid is impenetrable by X-rays, when an X-ray is taken the radiologist can see the outline of the colon.

biopsy

The process of obtaining human tissue so that it may be examined under a microscope by a pathologist. The tissue is obtained either by using a needle (needle biopsy) or by cutting out a section with a knife (excisional biopsy).

bronchoscopy

A procedure in which a fiber-optic instrument is passed through the mouth and down the trachea (windpipe) to examine the lung. Although the technology is similar to sigmoidoscopy and colonoscopy, the exam is technically more challenging because the natural response to having a tube introduced in your throat is either to gag or to swallow it (in which case the stomach would be examined).

cancer

In common usage, "a cellular tumor the natural course of which is fatal"; in practice, a diagnosis made on the size and shape of individual cells and the architecture of collections of cells.

carcinoma in situ

Cancer that involves only the cells in which it began and that has not spread to neighboring tissues.

CAT scan

Computerized axial tomography: an imaging procedure in which X-rays are manipulated in a computer to create a series of detailed pictures, viewable from different angles, of areas inside the body. Also called computerized tomography (CT scan).

colonoscopy

An examination of the entire colon using a fiber-optic scope.

colposcopy

A procedure in which the cervix is examined with an instrument inserted in the vagina.

control group

In a randomized trial, the group that does not receive the intervention being studied (either a test or a treatment). The control group typically receives conventional medical care, while the intervention group receives the test or treatment. Investigators compare the outcomes for the two groups to determine whether the intervention is better or worse than the conventional approach.

DCIS

Ductal carcinoma in situ: a tiny form of breast cancer involving a generally microscopic cancer that is confined to the breast ducts.

false positive

A test result that suggests cancer is present when it in fact is not. Also known as a "cancer scare."

fecal occult blood test

A screening test for colon cancer in which the patient spreads a small amount of stool onto a thin cardboard card. The card is sent to the laboratory where occult blood—blood not visible to the human eye—can be detected using a chemical reaction. Blood in the stool can be the result of many things, one of which is colon cancer.

fiber-optic scope

An instrument used to visualize the internal anatomy of hollow organs (e.g., stomach, colon, lungs). The long, flexible scope, containing thin strands of glass (or plastic) to transmit light, can even be directed around corners. The instrument also includes a number of tubes through which fluid (to wash off surfaces), air (to inflate the organ) and small surgical instruments (to biopsy worrisome tissue) can be passed.

five-year survival rate

Proportion of individuals diagnosed with cancer who are alive five years after diagnosis. Although this statistic is generally seen as reflecting the effectiveness of cancer treatment, it is greatly influenced by cancer testing. Five-year survival will increase whenever cancers are diagnosed earlier, even if the time of death is not postponed.

incidence

The rate of new cases of disease in a population; often calculated for a specific cancer (e.g., breast cancer incidence).

interval cancer

A cancer that becomes apparent in the period between two screening tests. Interval cancers tend to be particularly aggressive (fast growing).

intervention group

In a randomized trial, the group that receives the intervention being studied (either a test or a treatment). *See also* control group.

mammography

An X-ray exam of the breast. Used either as a screening test in women without symptoms of breast cancer or as a diagnostic test in women (and occasionally men) with a breast mass.

metastasis

The spread of cancer from one part of the body to distant sites in the body. Also the name given to the secondary tumor thus produced, a discrete collection of cancer cells that are separate from the original (primary) cancer.

metastasize   To spread from one part of the body to another.

metastatic   Having to do with metastasis.

morbidity   The amount of sickness or ill health in a population, excluding death. The term also encompasses the adverse effects of treatment. Morbidity and mortality combined thus become a comprehensive measure of population health.

mortality rate   The rate of death in a population; often calculated for a specific cancer (e.g., breast cancer mortality).

MRI   Magnetic resonance imaging: an imaging procedure in which a magnet linked to a computer is used to create detailed pictures of areas inside the body.

natural history   The natural course of an untreated disease.

needle biopsy   The removal of tissue or fluid with a needle for examination under a microscope.

Pap smear   A screening test for cervical cancer in which cells are collected from the cervix during a pelvic exam and examined under the microscope.

pathologist   A physician who specializes in examining human tissue under the microscope and who ultimately makes the diagnosis of cancer.

PET scan   Positron emission tomography scan: an imaging procedure that detects the metabolic activity of body tissues.

preclinical phase   The period of time that begins when a cell first becomes cancerous and ends when the cancer is large enough that it causes symptoms. The preclinical phase is thus the period during which a screening test could potentially detect the cancer.

PSA test   The blood test for prostate cancer; PSA stands for pros-
                            tate specific antigen.

pseudodisease   Cancers that never cause symptoms, either because
                            they don't grow at all or they grow so slowly that
                            people die of other causes before symptoms appear.

randomized trial   An experiment in which study participants are as-
                            signed to groups on the basis of chance. This is the best
                            way to ensure that study groups are similar and that dif-
                            ferences observed are the result of the experiment itself,
                            not of skewed population samples. *See also* control
                            group; intervention group.

relative risk   The ratio of one absolute risk to another. Relative risk
                            increases are typically expressed as percentages or fac-
                            tors (e.g., "20 percent higher" or "twice as high"). Rel-
                            ative risk decreases are typically expressed as a per-
                            centage reduction in absolute risk. For a person age 50
                            undergoing fecal occult blood testing, for example, the
                            relative risk of death from colon cancer is 33 percent
                            lower than for a similar-aged person who is not
                            screened (i.e., 2 per 1,000 vs. 3 per 1,000, or 33 percent
                            less). *See also* absolute risk.

sigmoidoscopy   A procedure in which a fiber-optic instrument is used
                            to examine the lower colon. Inserted into the rectum and
                            advanced partway up the colon, the instrument shines
                            light in both directions and can transmit images back to
                            a television monitor. The instrument also includes a
                            number of tubes through which fluid (to wash off sur-
                            faces), air (to inflate the colon), and small surgical in-
                            struments (to biopsy worrisome tissue) can be passed.

tissue   A group or layer of cells that are alike and that work to-
                            gether to perform a specific function.

tumor   An abnormal growth (mass of tissue) that is the prod-
                            uct of excessive cell division. Although in common us-
                            age often equated with cancer, a tumor may also be a
                            benign growth.

ultrasound   A technique employing a machine that sends and receives sound waves, much like a radar. Particularly good for distinguishing liquids from solids, it is used in the breast, heart (where it is typically called an echocardiogram), abdomen, and rectum (to examine the prostate).

NOTES

INTRODUCTION

1.   C. K. Meador, "The Last Well Person," *New England Journal of Medicine* 330 (1994): 440–441.

2.   These data come from the Center for Disease Control data collection effort on personal health behavior (it's called the Behavioral Risk Factor Surveillance System and involves more than 100,000 telephone surveys). Proportionally, these data translate to 60 percent of American men over age 50 being regularly tested for prostate cancer, 40 percent of men and women over age 50 being tested for colon cancer, 65 percent of women over age 40 being tested for breast cancer, and 85 percent of women over age 18 being tested for cervical cancer. See R. A. Smith, V. Cokkinides, and H. J. Eyre, "American Cancer Society Guidelines for Early Detection of Cancer," *CA: A Cancer Journal for Clinicians* 53 (2003): 27–43.

3.   This is my first (but by no means my last) oversimplification—because it turns out that the two issues are inexorably related. The answer about what to do if you know you have cancer depends in part on how it was found: cancers that cause symptoms are different from those found in people who are well.

4.   At first glance, it may be surprising that the typical 40-year-old woman is expected to die at a younger age (82) than the typical 80-year-old woman (89). When you think about it, however, you recognize that not all 40-year-olds survive to age 80, and those that do are healthier than average.

5.   Maureen Roberts is a physician who both ran one of the major randomized trials of mammography and had breast cancer herself (and ultimately died of it). See M. M. Roberts, "Breast Screening: Time for a Rethink?" *British Medical Journal* 299 (1989): 1153–1155.

CHAPTER 1

1. This is a simplified model of cancer. As I'll discuss in Chapter 3, just because an abnormality meets the cellular definition of cancer doesn't mean it will necessarily grow.

2. For an overall review of the mammography trials see K. Kerlikowske, D. Grady, S. M. Rubin, et al., "Efficacy of Screening Mammography," *JAMA* 273 (1995): 149–154. For a more critical review of the problems with various studies, see Chapter 9; also see O. Olsen and P. C. Gotzsche, "Cochrane Review on Screening for Breast Cancer with Mammography," *Lancet* 358 (2001): 1340–1342.

3. See B. P. Towler, L. Irwig, P. Glasziou, et al., "Screening for Colorectal Cancer Using the Faecal Occult Blood Test," *Cochrane Database of Systematic Reviews* 2000, no. 2.

4. There is a lot of interest in doing CAT scans of the chest to find early lung cancer, however. More on this later.

5. See L. Tabar, C. J. G. Fagerberg, M. C. South, et al., "The Swedish Two-County Trial of Mammographic Screening for Breast Cancer: Recent Results on Mortality and Tumor Characteristics," and L. Janzon and I. Andersson, "The Malmö Mammographic Screening Trial," both in *Cancer Screening*, ed. A. B. Miller, J. Chamberlain, N. E. Day, et al. (Sydney: Cambridge University Press, 1991); see esp. 32 (Fig. 5) and 41 (Table 6).

6. And there are other ways of saying the same thing: "9 in 1,000" could also be expressed as 0.009, 0.9 percent, or 1 in 111. Because there is some research that suggests that the "9 in 1,000" format is best understood, it is what I use here.

7. To be more precise, 9 in 1,000 is the estimated risk of death *without* screening. In fact, the national death index reflects a mixture of women, some of whom have had mammograms, some of whom have not. The actual percentage of women who have had mammograms is about 70 percent, according to the national health interview survey. Because we know the observed risk of death is a 70:30 blend of women (i.e., 70 percent who have vs. 30 percent who have not had mammography) and because we estimate that mammograms reduce the risk of death by a third, we can figure out (using a little algebra) the risk in each group. For more on baseline estimates of cancer risk, see S. Woloshin, L. M. Schwartz, and H. G. Welch, "Risk Charts: Putting Cancer in Context," *Journal of the National Cancer Institute* 94 (2002): 799–804.

8. See S. Shapiro, W. Venet, P. Strax, and L. Venet, *Periodic Screening for Breast Cancer: The Health Insurance Plan Project and Its Sequelae, 1963–1986* (Baltimore: John Hopkins University Press, 1988); and J. S. Mandel, J. H. Bond, T. R. Church, et al., "Reducing Mortality from Colorectal Cancer by Screening for Fecal Occult Blood: Minnesota Colon Cancer Control Study," *New England Journal of Medicine* 328 (1993): 1365–1371.

9. The differences between American and non-American studies are occasionally overblown. Witness the reaction of some American doctors to the disappointing findings of the Canadian trials of mammography, which might be paraphrased as "certainly there is nothing for us to learn from their work." They seemed to suggest that our colleagues to the north are working in some kind of third world country.

10. Because studies often have different follow-up periods (in this case 10 vs. 13 years) epidemiologists conventionally express death rates as the number of deaths per 1,000 people over 10 years of follow-up (which is also known as deaths per 10,000 person-years).

11. I must qualify this statement: I say it assuming that the patients excluded after randomization had no effect on the final result. Of course they might have. More on this in Chapter 9.

12. To be fair, they are obscured by the many who did not benefit.

CHAPTER 2

1. At the same time, the focus on ordering and discussing tests—which may have little to do with the patient's primary concern—can easily dominate a clinic visit. This may be one reason patients feel that their doctors no longer listen to them.

2. More precisely, most people will have negative screening tests most of the times they are tested. But as you'll see in a few pages, if you are tested every year for many years, the chance that you *always* have a negative test can get quite small.

3. L. G. Arnesson, B. Vitak, J. C. Manson, et al., "Diagnostic Outcome of Repeated Mammography Screening," *World Journal of Surgery* 19 (1995): 372–378; E. Lidbrink, J. Elfving, J. Frisell, and E. Jonsson, "Neglected Aspects of False Positive Findings of Mammography in Breast Cancer Screening: Analysis of False Positive Cases from the Stockholm Trial," *BMJ* 312 (1996): 273–276; and S. Ciatto, M. R. Del Turco, D. Giorgi, et al., "Assessment of Lesions Detected at Mammographic Screening: Performance at First or Repeat Screening in the Florence Programme," *Journal of Medical Screening* 1 (1994): 188–192.

4. K. Kerlikowske, D. Grady, J. Barclay, et al., "Positive Predictive Value of Screening Mammography by Age and Family History of Breast Cancer," *JAMA* 270 (1993): 2444–2450.

5. The reported false positive rates in the community have been between 8.5 and 11 percent. See S. P. Poplack, A. N. Tosteson, M. R. Grove, et al., "Mammography in 53,803 Women from the New Hampshire Mammography Network," *Radiology* 217 (2000): 832–840; H. G. Welch and E. S. Fisher, "Diagnostic Testing Following Screening Mammography in the Elderly," *Journal of the National*

Cancer Institute 90 (1998): 1389–1392; and M. L. Brown, F. Houn, E. A. Sickles, and L. G. Kessler, "Screening Mammography in Community Practice: Positive Predictive Value of Abnormal Findings and Yield of Follow-Up Diagnostic Procedures," *American Journal of Roentgenology* 165 (1995): 1373–1377.

6. *Abnormal* is defined as over 4.0 ng/ml; see E. D. Crawford, E. P. DeAntoni, R. Etzioni, et al., "Serum Prostate-Specific Antigen and Digital Rectal Examination for Early Detection of Prostate Cancer in a National Community-Based Program," *Urology* 47 (1996): 863–869.

7. See C. Mettlin, G. P. Murphy, R. J. Babaian, et al., "The Results of a Five-Year Early Prostate Cancer Detection Intervention," *Cancer* 77 (1996): 150–159; A. Reissigl, W. Horninger, K. Fink, et al., "Prostate Carcinoma Screening in the County of Tyrol, Austria," *Cancer* 80 (1997): 1818–1829; L. Maattanen, A. Auvinen, U. H. Stenman, et al., "European Randomized Study of Prostate Cancer Screening: First-Year Results of the Finnish Trial," *British Journal of Cancer* 79 (1999): 1210–1214; and L. Maattanen, A. Auvinen, U. H. Stenman, et al., "Three-Year Results of the Finnish Prostate Cancer Screening Trial," *Journal of the National Cancer Institute* 93 (2001): 552–553.

8. D. S. Smith, W. J. Catalona, and J. D. Herschman, "Longitudinal Screening for Prostate Cancer with Prostate Specific Antigen," *JAMA* 276 (1996): 1309–15.

9. That said, remember that PSA levels do tend to rise with age as the prostate enlarges. So some men who start with a normal PSA will develop abnormal PSA levels simply as a consequence of aging. The pattern of PSA elevation, however, is different in a slowly enlarging prostate than in an aggressive cancer: the former produces slowly rising levels that are slightly elevated, while the latter produces a rapid and dramatic elevation.

10. This assumes the specimens are rehydrated before testing—the recommended approach. See D. F. Ransohoff and C. A. Lang, "Screening for Colorectal Cancer with the Fecal Occult Blood Test: A Background Paper," *Annals of Internal Medicine* 126 (1997): 811–822.

11. S. L. Mount and J. L. Papillo, "A Study of 10,296 Pediatric and Adolescent Papanicolaou Smear Diagnoses in Northern New England," *Pediatrics* 103 (1999): 539–545. B. S. Sirovich, D. J. Gottlieb, E. S. Fisher, "The Burden of Prevention: Downstream Consequences of Pap Smear Testing in the Elderly," *Journal of Medical Screening* (in press).

12. Some might argue that such diagnoses are very necessary and that the treatment of these early abnormalities is the reason the death rate from cervical cancer has dropped so dramatically. Indeed, the drop is dramatic: cervical cancer mortality is one-fifth what it was 50 years ago. But many factors are at play in this change. And the number of ASCUS and SIL cases we are treating now far exceeds the number of cases of cervical cancer, even when it was much more frequent. Most of these abnormalities are simply not destined to become cervical cancer.

13.   Recommendations can be found in U.S. Preventive Services Task Force, *Guide to Clinical Preventive Services* (Baltimore: Williams & Wilkins, 1996), or at the Task Force web site, http://www.ahcpr.gov/clinic/uspstf/uspstopics.htm.

14.   J. G. Elmore, M. B. Barton, V. M. Moceri, et al., "Ten-Year Risk of False Positive Screening Mammograms and Clinical Breast Examinations," *New England Journal of Medicine* 338 (1998): 1089–1096.

15.   You might ask how the findings from 10 years of data collection compare with the back-of-the-envelope approach discussed previously. The two approaches in fact give remarkably similar results. The Pilgrim study reported a cumulative risk of 23.8 percent among women with a median of four mammograms and estimated a cumulative risk for 10 exams of 49.1 percent (using false positive probabilities observed at each round of screening). Given a 6.5 percent false positive rate, the back-of-the-envelope approach gives an estimate of 23.6 percent for four exams and 48.9 percent for 10.

16.   A. M. Kavanagh, G. Santow, and H. Mitchell, "Consequences of Current Patterns of Pap Smear and Colposcopy Use," *Journal of Medical Screening* 3 (1996): 29–34.

17.   J. S. Mandel, J. H. Bond, T. R. Church, et al., "Reducing Mortality from Colorectal Cancer by Screening for Fecal Occult Blood," *New England Journal of Medicine* 328 (1993): 1365–1371.

18.   The colonoscopy risk quoted here is from the randomized trial of fecal occult blood testing in the U.K.; see M. H. Robinson, J. D. Hardcastle, S. M. Moss, et al., "The Risks of Screening: Data from the Nottingham Randomized Controlled Trial of Faecal Occult Blood Screening for Colorectal Cancer," *Gut* 45 (1999): 588–92. Reported rates in the U.S. are considerably lower, but may underestimate what goes on in community practice. The bronchoscopy risk (see C. A. Pue and E. R. Pacht, "Complications of Fiberoptic Bronchoscopy at a University Hospital," *Chest* 107 [1995]: 430–32) reflects not simply the procedure but also the condition of the patients who receive it: smokers with bad lungs that are easily collapsed.

19.   I feel compelled to mention that I have tried to discourage this, but every year he goes to Florida for six months, and every year doctors there have persuaded him of the need for a biopsy.

20.   L. V. Rodriguez and M. K. Terris, "Risks and Complications of Transrectal Ultrasound Guided Prostate Needle Biopsy: A Prospective Study and Review of the Literature," *Journal of Urology* 160 (1998): 2115–2120.

21.   The medical terminology has been simplified; see W. J. Casarella, "A Patient's Viewpoint on a Current Controversy," *Radiology* 224 (2002): 927.

22.   C. Lerman, B. Trock, B. K. Rimer, et al., "Psychological and Behavioral Implications of Abnormal Mammograms," *Annals of Internal Medicine* 114 (1991): 657–661.

23.   H. G. Welch and E. S. Fisher, "Diagnostic Testing Following Screening

Mammography in the Elderly," *Journal of the National Cancer Institute* 90 (1998): 1389–1392.

CHAPTER 3

1.   It is not, however, unheard of. In fact, many books written by physicians include accounts of similar cases. See, for example, Bernie S. Siegel, *Love, Medicine, and Miracles: Lessons Learned about Self-Healing from a Surgeon's Experience with Exceptional Patients* (New York: Harper Perennial, 1990).

2.   *Rare* is, of course, a relative term. Neuroblastoma is rare relative to any of the familiar adult cancers (e.g., lung, colon, prostate, breast). On the other hand, neuroblastoma is second only to leukemia in terms of the leading cancers in children (who, as a group, rarely get cancer).

3.   F. Bessho, "Effects of Mass Screening on Age-Specific Incidence of Neuroblastoma," *International Journal of Cancer* 67 (1996): 520–522.

4.   F. Bessho, "Where Should Neuroblastoma Mass Screening Go?" *Lancet* 348 (1996): 1672.

5.   K. Yamamoto, R. Hanada, A. Kikuchi, et al., "Spontaneous Regression of Localized Neuroblastoma Detected by Mass Screening," *Journal of Clinical Oncology* 16 (1998): 1265–1269.

6.   I use the term *tumor* instead of *cancer* because many of these were not biopsied; all had the radiological appearance of cancer, however, and those that were biopsied were diagnosed as cancer. See M. A. Bosniak, B. A. Birnbaum, G. A. Krinsky, and J. Waisman, "Small Renal Parenchymal Neoplasms: Further Observations on Growth," *Radiology* 197 (1995): 589–597.

7.   The Tennessee cases are reported in D. L. Page, W. D. Dupont, L. W. Rogers, et al., "Continued Local Recurrence of Carcinoma 15–25 Years after a Diagnosis of Low Grade Ductal Carcinoma In Situ of the Breast Treated Only by Biopsy," *Cancer* 76 (1995): 1197–1200. The Italian cases are in V. Eusebi, M. P. Foschini, M. G. Cook, et al., "Long-Term Follow-up of In Situ Carcinoma of the Breast with Special Emphasis on Clinging Carcinoma," *Seminars in Diagnostic Pathology* 6 (1989): 165–173.

8.   M. D. Lagios, F. R. Margolin, P. R. Westdahl, and M. R. Rose, "Mammographically Detected Ductal Carcinoma In Situ: Frequency of Local Recurrence following Tylectomy and Prognostic Effect of Nuclear Grade on Local Reoccurrence," *Cancer* 63 (1989): 618–624.

9.   The fastest case appeared three years after biopsy. This suggests that when DCIS progresses, it progresses so slowly that the transformation to invasive cancer would be "caught" by a repeat mammogram. This is a situation where many patients might rationally choose a follow-up test over aggressive therapy such as mastectomy or radiation.

10.   V. L. Ernster, J. Barclay, K. Kerlikowske, et al., "Mortality among Women with Ductal Carcinoma In Situ of the Breast in the Population-Based Surveillance, Epidemiology, and End Results Program," *Archives of Internal Medicine* 160 (2000): 953–958.

11.   J. H. Wasson, D. J. Reda, R. C. Bruskewitz, et al., "A Comparison of Transurethral Surgery with Watchful Waiting for Moderate Symptoms of Benign Prostatic Hyperplasia: The Veterans Affairs Cooperative Study Group on Transurethral Resection of the Prostate," *New England Journal of Medicine* 332 (1995): 75–79.

12.   Since the urethra—the tube that connects the bladder to the opening of the penis—runs through the prostate, an enlarged prostate tends to compress this tube, making it more difficult to urinate.

13.   SEER is the federal government's primary effort to collect and report on cancer incidence, initial treatment, and survival. This database includes information from cancer registries in the states of Connecticut, Iowa, New Mexico, Utah, and Hawaii and the metropolitan areas of Detroit, San Francisco, Seattle–Puget Sound, and Atlanta. Together these areas represent approximately 10 percent of the U.S. population.

14.   Some may be interested in why there was a sharp drop following the sharp rise. One explanation is biological: when the PSA was first used, it identified many preexisting cases of prostate cancer that were lurking below the surface. In the ensuing years, these preexisting cases were no longer there to be found—instead new cases had to develop. The other explanation is sociological: physicians were caught off guard by how much prostate cancer could be found in elderly men and subsequently directed the test more prudently toward men who had a longer life expectancy (and less cancer). The truth likely involves both explanations.

15.   Several randomized trials of prostate cancer screening are ongoing, although no results have yet been published. One of the biggest is the PLCO trial, which is studying screening not only for prostate cancer (P), but also for lung, colorectal, and ovarian cancer (LCO).

16.   See A. L. Potosky, J. Legler, P. C. Albertsen, et al., "Health Outcomes after Prostatectomy or Radiotherapy for Prostate Cancer: Results from the Prostate Cancer Outcomes Study," *Journal of the National Cancer Institute* 92 (2000): 1582–1592.

17.   See P. C. Albertsen, D. G. Fryback, B. E. Storer, et al., "Long-Term Survival among Men with Conservatively Treated Localized Prostate Cancer," *JAMA* 274 (1995): 626–631. "Low-grade" is the pathologists' description of how aggressive the cancer appears under the microscope. Some men in this study received hormonal therapy.

18.   Two possible approaches stand out. First, PSA testing could be directed at younger men, in whom pseudodisease is much less of a problem. To some extent this is happening already. Second, the definition of an abnormal test might be changed, which in turn would alter the frequency at which men undergo biop-

sies. What are now considered moderately elevated values—that lead to biopsy—for example, might be rechecked in three months, with biopsies performed only if the PSA rose further.

19.   H. Tulinius, "Latent Malignancies at Autopsy: A Little-Used Source of Information on Cancer Biology," in *Autopsy in Epidemiology and Medical Research*, ed. E. Riboli and M. Delendi (Lyon: International Agency for Research on Cancer, 1991).

20.   See J. E. Montie, D. P. Wood, J. E. Pontes, et al., "Adenocarcinoma of the Prostate in Cystoprostatectomy Specimens Removed for Bladder Cancer," *Cancer* 63 (1989): 381–385. Note that the removal of a cancerous bladder includes removing the prostate—providing the pathologist the opportunity to examine a prostate not known to be diseased. Because prostate and bladder cancer are not believed to be related, this analysis contributes to the estimation of the underlying reservoir in the general population.

21.   In this study, the pathologists examined the prostate every 5 mm—the equivalent of about 10 tissue slices per prostate (the typical prostate being about 50 mm long). If they had taken slices every 2 mm (i.e., examined 25 slices), they might have found more cancer—as you'll see in the next chapter.

CHAPTER 4

1.   You might be surprised that hoarseness can be a symptom of lung cancer. The nerve to the vocal cords loops down into the chest near the lymph nodes that drain the lung. Lung cancer often involves these nodes, which in turn enlarge and trap the nerve. That can paralyze the vocal cords, causing hoarseness.

2.   Because the lungs are longer in the back than the front, all chest CAT scans have to include some of the abdomen if they are going to include the entire lung.

3.   Whether it was good or bad luck is very hard to know. It certainly is not clear what should happen next for this patient—as I'll come back to in Chapter 8.

4.   What the physical exam can and cannot detect, of course, depends on many factors. Among them are the precise location of the cancer, the size of the patient (it's easier to feel things in thin people), the experience of the physician, and the amount of effort given to the exam.

5.   A. R. Spouge, S. R. Wilson, and B. Wooley, "Abdominal Sonography in Asymptomatic Executives: Prevalence of Pathologic Findings, Potential Benefits, and Problems," *Journal of Ultrasound Medicine* 15 (1996): 763–767.

6.   You may be wondering why, in a kidney transplant, these researchers used ultrasound, CAT scans, and needle biopsies rather than examining tissue sections from the removed kidney. The reason is that the native kidneys are routinely left inside the body; the new kidney is simply added, low in the pelvis.

7.   See J. D. Doublet, M. N. Peraldi, B. Gattegno, et al., "Renal Cell Carcinoma of Native Kidneys: Prospective Study of 129 Renal Transplant Patients," *Journal of Urology* 158 (1997): 42–44; I. Ishikawa, "Renal Cell Carcinoma in Chronic Hemodialysis Patients—a 1990 Questionnaire Study in Japan," *Kidney International: Supplement* 41 (1993): S167–169; and A. C. Gulanikar, P. P. Daily, N. K. Kilambi, et al., "Prospective Pretransplant Ultrasound Screening in 206 Patients for Acquired Renal Cysts and Renal Cell Carcinoma," *Transplantation* 66 (1998): 1669–1672.

8.   I say this because the risk elevation is many times that typically identified in rigorous epidemiological studies of cancer risk factors. The classic "really big" risk factor is smoking for lung cancer—about a 10- to 15-fold increase in risk over nonsmokers, and even higher for heavy smokers. Simply having lung failure (chronic lung disease), on the other hand, is a relatively small risk factor for lung cancer. I suspect that kidney failure is a similarly small risk factor for kidney cancer.

9.   Although patients were enrolled in the late 1970s and early 1980s, follow-up has continued for many years. See R. S. Fontana, "Screening for Lung Cancer," in *Screening for Cancer,* ed. A. B. Miller (Orlando, Fla.: Academic Press, 1985), 377–395; and P. M. Marcus, E. J. Bergstralh, R. M. Fagerstrom, et al., "Lung Cancer Mortality in the Mayo Lung Project: Impact of Extended Follow-up," *Journal of the National Cancer Institute* 92 (2000): 1308–1316.

10.   W. C. Black, "Overdiagnosis: An Underrecognized Cause of Confusion and Harm in Cancer Screening," *Journal of the National Cancer Institute* 92 (2000): 1280–1282.

11.   S. Sone, S. Takashima, F. Li, et al., "Mass Screening for Lung Cancer with Mobile Spiral Computed Tomography Scanner," *Lancet* 351 (1998): 1242–1245.

12.   The word *typical* obscures the fact that there is a broad range of prostate size. The volume given here is based on a gland 4 cm in diameter, which is somewhat smaller than average. Thus, the proportion of the gland examined is probably overestimated.

13.   P. M. Arnold, T. H. Niemann, and R. R. Bahnson, "Extended Sector Biopsy for Detection of Carcinoma of the Prostate," *Urologic Oncology* 6 (2001): 91–93.

14.   N. Fleshner and L. Klotz, "Role of 'Saturation Biopsy' in the Detection of Prostate Cancer among Difficult Diagnostic Cases," *Urology* 60 (2002): 93–97.

15.   These data come from the U.S. Medicare program and reflect the experience of patients most likely to have these cancers: those age 65 and older. Younger patients would be expected to have lower operative mortality. See E. V. Finlayson and J. D. Birkmeyer, "Operative Mortality with Elective Surgery in Older Adults," *Effective Clinical Practice* 4 (2001): 172–177.

16.   For the Canadian study, see W. G. Woods, R. N. Gao, J. J. Shuster, et al., "Screening of Infants and Mortality Due to Neuroblastoma," *New England Journal of Medicine* 346 (2002): 1041–1046; for the German study, see F. H. Schilling,

C. Spix, F. Berthold, et al., "Neuroblastoma Screening at One Year of Age," *New England Journal of Medicine* 346 (2002): 1047–1053.

17.   More precisely, the incidence of neuroblastoma was twice as high among children screened as among children in the general population. For details on how the expected incidence was obtained in the Canadian study, see W. G. Woods, M. Tuchman, L. L. Robison, et al., "A Population-Based Study of the Usefulness of Screening for Neuroblastoma," *Lancet* 348 (1996): 1682–1687.

18.   See M. J. McFarlane, A. R. Feinstein, and C. K. Wells, "Clinical Features of Lung Cancers Discovered as a Postmortem 'Surprise,' " *Chest* 90 (1986): 520–523; and C. K. Chan, C. K. Wells, M. J. McFarlane, and A. R. Feinstein, "More Lung Cancer but Better Survival: Implications of Secular Trends in 'Necropsy Surprise' Rates," *Chest* 96 (1989): 291–296.

19.   Pathologists generally do have some clue about where to look for cancer: they might feel a mass or be directed to it by an X-ray. But when they are trying to define how much cancer people without symptoms have, they really don't know precisely where to look. This is also true in a few clinical examples, such as searching for cancer in lymph nodes that look normal to the naked eye or random needle biopsies of the prostate.

20.   H. R. Harach, K. O. Franssila, and V. M. Wasenius, "Occult Papillary Carcinoma of the Thyroid: A 'Normal' Finding in Finland. A Systematic Autopsy Study," *Cancer* 56 (1985): 531–538. The autopsies were consecutive, which means every time an autopsy was performed in the hospital the researchers did a systematic exam of the thyroid. Thus, the subjects were not selected for some unusual quality; rather, they were largely older Finns who died in the hospital.

21.   This dramatic rise was first brought to the attention of doctors in 1996. See V. L. Ernster, J. Barclay, K. Kerlikowske, et al., "Incidence of and Treatment for Ductal Carcinoma In Situ of the Breast," *JAMA* 275 (1996): 913–918.

22.   In Figure 9, the predicted incidence of invasive cancer is calculated by assuming all DCIS progresses to invasive cancer in an average of three years. The value for a specific year in the line titled "Expected incidence of late-stage cancer assuming total cancer incidence is stable" is the average invasive incidence observed in the mid-1970s (100 per 100,000) *minus* the DCIS incidence three years earlier (e.g. to calculate what was expected in 1980, the 1977 DCIS rate is used). The value for a specific year in the line titled "Expected incidence of late-stage cancer assuming total cancer incidence is rising" is the predicted incidence of the specified year (where the prediction is based at 100 per 100,000 in 1973 and increases 1 percent per year) *minus* the DCIS incidence three years earlier.

23.   H. G. Welch and W. C. Black, "Using Autopsy Series to Estimate the Disease 'Reservoir' for Ductal Carcinoma In Situ of the Breast: How Much More Breast Cancer Can We Find?" *Annals of Internal Medicine* 127 (1997): 1023–1028. The first four studies represent women who died in the hospital, were not known to have

had breast cancer during life, and had a surprise case diagnosed during an autopsy (these are analogous to the Yale–New Haven autopsy study that identified surprise cases of lung cancer). The last three studies are forensic autopsies: consecutive deaths being investigated by a coroner (i.e., deaths in which homicide is suspected).

24.   And there is even more potential to find "precancers." Some of the studies also included information on breast abnormalities believed to be cancer precursors. Typically, a third of all women studied would have evidence of "atypical hyperplasia," "severe hyperplasia," "marked intraductal hyperplasia," or "atypical ductal hyperplasia"—all worrisome findings because they might become cancer. Still, the more there is, the more the abnormality should be considered "normal."

CHAPTER 5

1.   S. L. Robbins and R. S. Cotran, *The Pathologic Basis of Disease,* 3d ed. (Philadelphia: W. B. Saunders Co., 1984), 265. Although the passage disappeared from later editions, the notion still applies.

2.   I want to thank two of our pathologists, Nora Ratcliffe and Alan Schned, for sharing multiple images of prostate disease with me and explaining some of the daily distinctions they are asked to make.

3.   C. K. Allam, D. G. Bostwick, J. A. Hayes, et al., "Interobserver Variability in the Diagnosis of High-Grade Prostatic Intraepithelial Neoplasia and Adenocarcinoma," *Modern Pathology* 9 (1996): 742–751.

4.   For simplicity, the word *cancer* here combines the diagnoses of "cancer" and "suspicious for cancer." The authors also chose to combine these diagnoses in some of their analyses. Lumping diagnoses together makes agreement more likely (that is, if three pathologists say suspicious for cancer and five say cancer, they are all said to be in agreement).

5.   J. I. Epstein, D. J. Grignon, P. A. Humphrey, et al., "Interobserver Reproducibility in the Diagnosis of Prostatic Intraepithelial Neoplasia," *American Journal of Surgical Pathology* 19 (1995): 873–886.

6.   Using cases "selected to represent the full diagnostic spectrum" probably makes agreement less likely, since that makes for a higher incidence of rare diagnoses than in real life.

7.   As with the prior study, the word *cancer* here combines two diagnoses, in this case "cancer" and "cannot rule out cancer." Again, this lumping makes agreement more likely. To be more precise about the specimen for which they all agree, for example, five pathologists diagnosed cancer while two said they could not rule out cancer.

8.   E. R. Farmer, R. Gonin, and M. P. Hanna, "Discordance in the Histopatho-
logic Diagnosis of Melanoma and Melanocytic Nevi between Expert Pathologists,"
Human Pathology 27 (1996): 528–531.

9.   S. J. Schnitt, J. L. Connolly, F. A. Tavassoli, et al., "Interobserver Reproducibility in the Diagnosis of Ductal Proliferative Breast Lesions Using Standardized Criteria," *American Journal of Surgical Pathology* 16 (1992):1133–1143.

10.   Even pathologists find it difficult to describe the cancer vs. noncancer
distinction—one, for example, wrote that severe ductal atypia "is similar to DCIS,
although the pathologic alterations of the former are somewhat less marked" (C. E.
Alpers and S. R. Wellings, "The Prevalence of Carcinoma In Situ in Normal and
Cancer-associated Breasts," *Human Pathology* 16 [1985]: 797).

11.   W. A. Wells, P. A. Carney, M. S. Eliassen, et al., "Statewide Study of Diagnostic Agreement in Breast Pathology," *Journal of the National Cancer Institute* 90
(1998): 142–145.

12.   Since there was agreement in 8 of 16 cases, that means there was disagreement about the remaining 8. Let me tell you about them: in one case one
pathologist said no cancer, the other 25 said yes; and in seven cases, one pathologist said cancer, the others said no. But the one pathologist was almost always a
different individual, suggesting an element of random error.

13.   I purposely avoid being too precise here. These numbers are, of course,
also affected by how many pathologists are asked to examine the slides (8 in the
VA prostate cancer study, 26 in the New Hampshire mammography study). As
more pathologists are involved, disagreement becomes more likely. So while on
first glance one might surmise that disagreement is more likely in breast cancer
than in prostate cancer, I don't think we really know.

CHAPTER 6

1.   The whole idea of scheduled health maintenance, in fact, started with routine vaccination of children.

2.   Before doing an X-ray test that involves an injection of dye, for example,
we do a test to make sure the kidneys are functioning properly.

3.   Generally, the more abnormalities (such as polyps) that are found, the
stronger the case for a repeat colonoscopy and the stronger the case for a shorter
interval (e.g., three years instead of 10). But when it comes to specifics, we are only
guessing (e.g., should the interval be three years? one year? 10 years? or six
months?).

4.   Although my focus here is on how health maintenance can compete with
problems patients want doctors to attend to, testing can also distract from other
problems that physicians should attend to. In particular, I am thinking about the
need for doctors to continually reassess the appropriateness of previous diagnoses

and the usefulness of previously prescribed medications. This can be a laborious task. If it doesn't happen, however, the medical care can act like a one-way valve, the result being more testing, more diagnoses, more medications.

5.   The length of a typical clinic visit is not the result of any specific administrative decision, instead it is the product of counterbalancing forces. Doctors in private practice earn more, the more patients they see in a day. But patients are less satisfied if they feel shortchanged on time. Salaried doctors are generally told how many patients they are expected to see in a day (often based on private-sector rates) and they allot their time accordingly. For time trends on the length of clinic visits, see D. Mechanic, D. D. McAlpine, and M. Rosenthal, "Are Patients' Office Visits with Physicians Getting Shorter?" *New England Journal of Medicine* 344 (2001): 198–204.

CHAPTER 7

1.   One study found that physicians' estimates of the risk of being sued was three times the actual rate. See A. G. Lawthers, A. R. Localio, N. M. Laird, et al., "Physicians' Perception of the Risk of Being Sued," *Journal of Health Politics and Policy Law* 17 (1992): 463–482.

2.   The meeting is called M & M, which stands for morbidity and mortality. This reflects its historical focus: patients who had suffered harm or who had died during their hospitalization. We have expanded the focus, however, to include patients whose diagnosis and/or treatment was complex or that raise general issues with which the medical staff deal frequently.

3.   See B. J. Hillman, C. A. Joseph, M. R. Mabry, et al., "Frequency and Costs of Diagnostic Imaging in Office Practice—A Comparison of Self-Referring and Radiologist-Referring Physicians," *New England Journal of Medicine* 323 (1990): 1604–1608.

4.   As early as 1971, Richard Nixon said that the traditional health care system "operates episodically" with an "illogical incentive" that rewards illness. See Paul Starr, *The Social Transformation of American Medicine* (New York: Basic Books, 1982), 396.

5.   For example, the National Committee for Quality Assurance, perhaps the best-known source of information on quality, uses both the proportion of women receiving Pap smears and the proportion receiving mammograms as measures of quality.

6.   To be fair, there are people who are working to develop quality measures for the care of the sick. Unfortunately, these are much more difficult to devise; specifically, it is difficult to identify measures that are both sufficiently broad (i.e., apply to more than a handful of a doctor's patients), so that a doctor can be reliably measured, and sufficiently precise (i.e., detail the patients' presenting char-

acteristics, such as age, blood pressure, medications, and conditions), so that there is little ambiguity about what constitutes a "high quality" course of action.

7.   At this point you might reasonably wonder about my motivation for writing this book. Not surprisingly, I am motivated by multiple factors. Professional and public recognition is surely one. Another is more mundane: having a solid product to justify a sabbatical; and another more personal: to emulate my father. But these are generic motivations to write a book—any book. I really did want to write this book, both because the topic has been my primary concern for the past decade and because I believe the general public has been exposed to only one side of cancer testing; I wanted to try to communicate the other side.

8.   Although I remember much of the story as it unfolded, I am indebted to Suzanne Fletcher for putting it down on paper. See S. W. Fletcher, "Whither Scientific Deliberation in Health Policy Recommendations? Alice in the Wonderland of Breast Cancer Screening," *New England Journal of Medicine* 336 (1997): 1180–1183.

9.   While breast cancer is less common in younger women, the problem of pseudodisease is actually more common. The panel did not quantify the problem of pseudodisease because that's hard to do. They did say that one of every eight biopsies in this age group is read as DCIS, the diagnosis most likely to be pseudodisease. The biopsy rate varies depending on who reads the mammograms. But a ballpark estimate is that for every 1,000 40-year-old women screened over 10 years, somewhere between 10 and 20 will be diagnosed with breast cancer unnecessarily.

10.   I'm afraid this is getting close to standard behavior. A few years later the American College of Radiology immediately dismissed the results of probably the most carefully done study of mammography to date. The same day the study appeared in the *Journal of the National Cancer Institute,* the college was issuing press releases and urging its members (radiologists) to write letters—a template was provided—to the editor of their local paper.

11.   See G. Kolata, "Stand on Mammograms Greeted by Outrage," *New York Times,* January 28, 1997, C1; and G. Kolata, "Mammogram Talks Prove Indefinite," *New York Times,* January 24, 1997, A1.

CHAPTER 8

1.   Although occasionally patients with kidney cancer will have only part of a kidney removed, the most common practice is to remove the whole thing. Since so much fluid circulates through the kidney (both blood and urine), cutting away a portion often leads to fluid accumulation and leaks. Because most of us can do well with just one kidney, taking the whole thing actually leads to fewer problems.

2.   For a simple summary of the operative mortality following specific pro-

cedures in older adults, see E. V. A. Finlayson and J. D. Birkmeyer, "Operative Mortality with Elective Surgery in Older Adults," *Effective Clinical Practice* 4 (2001): 172–177. Now some of these procedures may be done using a "minimally invasive" technique that probably leads to lower mortality.

3.   All three of the statistics discussed here—incidence, mortality, and five-year survival—are publicly available thanks to the federal government's SEER (Surveillance, Epidemiology, and End Results) program. Data for all the major cancers for each year starting in 1973 can be found at http://seer.cancer.gov.

4.   A rate of 3 per 100,000 makes this a rare cause of cancer death. For perspective, the mortality rate for colon cancer is about 17 per 100,000, and lung cancer about 50 per 100,000.

5.   For more on how mortality (as well as incidence and five-year survival) is age-adjusted, see the appendix at the end of the chapter.

6.   United Press International Wire Report, "Gore Faults GOP on Cancer Effort," August 10, 1999.

7.   Congressional Record, Kay Bailey Hutchinson Statement on National Breast Cancer Survivors' Day (Senate–April 1, 1998), 105th Congress, S3009.

8.   See T. Blair, "Britain's Treatment of Cancer Just Isn't Good Enough," *Daily Mail* (London), May 20, 1999, 5; and I. Murray, "Blair Plan Aims to Cut Cancer Deaths by Fifth," *Times* (London), May 21, 1999.

9.   Five-year survival is not, however, a good measure for a randomized trial of a cancer screening test. In this case, people without cancer are invited to join the study. Because one group gets tested and the other group does not, the five-year survival clock is necessarily started at different times in the two groups, making comparison impossible.

10.   For more on national trends in five-year survival and their lack of relationship to cancer mortality, see H. G. Welch, L. M. Schwartz, and S. Woloshin, "Are Increasing 5-Year Survival Rates Evidence of Success against Cancer?" *JAMA* 283 (2000): 2975–2978.

11.   M. Dunlop, "2 Studies Conflict on When to Test for Breast Cancer," *Toronto Star,* October 24, 1992, A11.

12.   The UCLA study is K. H. Tsui, O. Shvarts, R. B. Smith, et al., "Renal Cell Carcinoma: Prognostic Significance of Incidentally Detected Tumors," *Journal of Urology* 163 (2000):426–430; the Cornell study is C. I. Henschke, D. I. McCauley, D. F. Yankelevitz, et al., "Early Lung Cancer Action Project: Overall Design and Findings from Baseline Screening," *Lancet* 354 (1999): 99–105.

13.   G. Kolata, "Large Study Urged for New Method of Detecting Lung Cancer," *New York Times,* October 27, 1999, A19.

14.   See Chapter 4 and S. Sone, S. Takashima, F. Li, et al., "Mass Screening for Lung Cancer with Mobile Spiral Computed Tomography Scanner," *Lancet* 351 (1998): 1242–1245.

15.   The latest statistics can be found at http://seer.cancer.gov. Go to Cancer Statistics Review 1973–[latest year] and locate the most recent issue; click on Section I overview and find "SEER Incidence and US Mortality Trends, 1950–[latest year]."

16.   In the case of breast cancer, some of the observed increase in incidence is undoubtedly real, given the increasing tendency of women to delay childbirth or remain childless. One of the best-understood risk factors for breast cancer is a woman's history of hormonal cycling: earlier menarche (onset of periods), older age at first pregnancy, childlessness, and late menopause all increase the risk of breast cancer. (Although even here, the increased risk is small relative to that associated with BRCA, the so-called breast cancer gene.)

17.   To their credit, it is a problem that dermatologists themselves recognize. See R. A. Swerlick and S. Chen, "The Melanoma Epidemic: More Apparent than Real?" *Mayo Clinic Proceedings* 72 (1997): 559–564.

18.   Some primary care practitioners also do skin biopsies. This is in part because they are a service to patients, in part because they are fun to do, and in part because they are billable procedures.

19.   I have pieced the story together from several sources. See D. F. Austin, P. J. Reynolds, M. A. Snyder, et al., "Malignant Melanoma among Employees at Lawrence Livermore National Laboratory," *Lancet* 2 (1981): 712–716; R. A. Hiatt and B. Fireman, "The Possible Effect of Increased Surveillance on the Incidence of Malignant Melanoma," *Preventive Medicine* 15 (1986): 652–660; and G. Gong, A. S. Whittemore, D. West, and D. H. Moore, "Cutaneous Melanoma at the Lawrence Livermore National Laboratory: Comparison with Rates in Two San Francisco Bay Area Counties," *Cancer Causes Control* 3 (1992): 191–197.

20.   "High Melanoma Rate Found in Children near Lab," *Los Angeles Times,* October 15, 1995, A29.

21.   From 1950 to 2000, stomach cancer mortality has fallen 83 percent, cervix 79 percent, uterus 69 percent, testis 73 percent, and Hodgkin's disease 75 percent. See http://seer.cancer.gov.

22.   From 1950 to 2000, head and neck cancer mortality has fallen 50 percent, thyroid 45 percent, and bladder 31 percent. See http://seer.cancer.gov.

23.   H. G. Welch and W. C. Black, "Are Deaths within 1 Month of Cancer-directed Surgery Attributed to Cancer?" *Journal of the National Cancer Institute* 94 (2002): 1066–1070.

CHAPTER 9

1.   Let me elaborate a bit on randomized trials. First, not everybody who wants to participate is necessarily able to. Randomized trials generally have en-

try criteria that determine eligibility. For a screening test, the criteria are broad: participants must fall within a specified age range (e.g., between 40 and 70) and have no prior history of the cancer being tested for. Second, randomized trials often involve more than two groups. Some treatment studies have randomized patients into as many as six groups.

2.   See S. Shapiro, W. Venet, P. Strax, and L. Venet, *Periodic Screening for Breast Cancer: The Health Insurance Plan Project and Its Sequelae, 1963–1986* (Baltimore: Johns Hopkins University Press, 1988).

3.   See M. M. Roberts, F. E. Alexander, T. J. Anderson, et al., "Edinburgh Trial of Screening for Breast Cancer: Mortality at Seven Years," *Lancet* 335 (1990): 241–246.

4.   See L. Nystrom, L. E. Rutqvist, S. Wall, et al., "Breast Cancer Screening with Mammography: Overview of Swedish Randomized Trials," *Lancet* 341 (1993): 973–978.

5.   See A. B. Miller, C. J. Baines, T. To, and C. Wall, "Canadian National Breast Screening Study: 1. Breast Cancer Detection and Death Rates among Women Aged 40 to 49 Years," *Canadian Medical Association Journal* 147 (1992): 1459–1476; and idem, "Canadian National Breast Screening Study: 2. Breast Cancer Detection and Death Rates among Women Aged 50–59 Years," *Canadian Medical Association Journal* 147 (1992): 1477–1488.

6.   As women entered the trial, a study nurse asked about breast symptoms (i.e., nipple discharge, lumps, pain) and performed a clinical breast exam. Those women who they thought might have cancer were excluded from the study and referred directly for a diagnostic mammogram. The allegation was that at the same time the nurses might also have identified women with a high risk of breast cancer and directed them to the mammography group. For more on the allegation, see D. B. Kopans and S. A. Feig, "The Canadian National Breast Screening Study: A Critical Review," *American Journal of Roentgenology* 161 (1993): 755–760; and N. F. Boyd, R. A. Jong, M. J. Yaffe, et al., "A Critical Appraisal of the Canadian National Breast Cancer Screening Study," *Radiology* 189 (1993): 661–663.

7.   Reuters, "Cancer Study to Be Reviewed," *Toronto Star,* February 15, 1995, A4.

8.   J. C. Bailar and B. MacMahon, "Randomization in the Canadian National Breast Screening Study: A Review for Evidence of Subversion," *Canadian Medical Association Journal* 156 (1997): 193–199.

9.   H. Seiden, "How Critics See Breast Cancer Study: Is This a War of Science or Simply Dirty Politics?" *Toronto Star,* December 10, 1992, C5.

10.   C. J. Baines, "The Canadian National Breast Screening Study: A Perspective on Criticisms," *Annals of Internal Medicine* 120 (1994): 326–334; and S. A. Narod, "On Being the Right Size: A Reappraisal of Mammography Trials in Canada and Sweden," *Lancet* 349 (1997): 1846.

11.   The group is named after Archie Cochrane (1909–1988), a British med-

ical researcher who advocated rigorous testing of the effectiveness of medical interventions. His book *Effectiveness and Efficiency: Random Reflections on Health Services* (1972) is short, simple, and arguably one of the most influential books in medicine.

12.   O. Olsen and P. C. Gotzsche, "Cochrane Review on Screening for Breast Cancer with Mammography," *Lancet* 358 (2001): 1340–1342. In addition, a 100-plus-page supporting document is available at http://image.thelancet.com/lancet/extra/fullreport.pdf. The *New York Times* article, "Study Sets Off Debate over Mammograms' Value," by G. Kolata, appeared on page 1A of the December 9, 2001, edition.

13.   Shapiro et al., *Periodic Screening for Breast Cancer.*

14.   L. Nystrom, I. Andersson, N. Bjurstam, et al., "Long-Term Effects of Mammography Screening: Updated Overview of the Swedish Randomised Trials," *Lancet* 359 (2002): 909–919.

15.   See P. C. Gotzsche and O. Olsen, "Is Screening for Breast Cancer with Mammography Justifiable?" *Lancet* 355 (2000): 129.

16.   The 10,000 figure is a crude estimate: there are 14,000 radiologists in the United States, not all of whom read mammograms.

17.   The biggest effect of screening observed in the Canadian studies was that more DCIS was found in women receiving mammography. In Canada 1, 71 women were diagnosed with DCIS in the mammography group as compared to 29 women in the usual care group; in Canada 2 the corresponding figures were 71 and 16. In neither study did women appear to benefit from early cancer detection, even after more than 10 years of follow-up. See A. B. Miller, T. To, C. J. Baines, and C. Wall, "The Canadian National Breast Screening Study-1: Breast Cancer Mortality after 11 to 16 Years of Follow-up. A Randomized Screening Trial of Mammography in Women Age 40 to 49 Years," *Annals of Internal Medicine* 137 (2002): 305–312; and idem, "Canadian National Breast Screening Study-2: 13-Year Results of a Randomized Trial in Women Aged 50–59 Years," *Journal of the National Cancer Institute* 92 (2000): 1490–1499.

18.   At this point, typically, a mammogram is ordered. Now, however, it is a diagnostic test, not a screening test.

19.   Breast tissue and many breast cancers are influenced by sex hormones. Estrogen probably causes some breast cancers to start and certainly leads many others to grow faster. Antiestrogens—like Tamoxifen—are increasingly used both to treat breast cancer and to prevent it.

20.   The statisticians arrive at this number by performing what is known as a sample size calculation. It is an effort to address an unfortunate fact: a study may miss an effect that really exists simply by chance. If a study has few participants, the chance is high. If it has a large number, the chance is low. The researchers have to decide what level of chance is acceptable and the size of the effect they want to be sure not to miss. The statistician then uses a rather involved

formula (usually now part of a software package) to determine how many patients need to be studied.

In case you *are* a statistician, you will want to know that all sample size calculations are based on a two-sided alpha error of 0.05 and have a power of 90 percent.

21.   If we want to know about right position for some of those dials (e.g. two- vs. three-view mammography, or annual vs. biennial spiral CAT scan), we will need to take into account these smaller effects.

22.   See Early Breast Cancer Trialists' Collaborative Group, "Favourable and Unfavourable Effects on Long-Term Survival of Radiotherapy for Early Breast Cancer: An Overview of the Randomised Trials," *Lancet* 355 (2000): 1757–1770; and J. F. Boivin, "Second Cancers and Other Late Side Effects of Cancer Treatment. A Review," *Cancer* 65, no. 3 (suppl.) (1990): 770–775.

23.   Patients were diagnosed with cancer between 1973 and 1987. See B. W. Brown, C. Brauner, and M. C. Minnotte, "Noncancer Deaths in White Adult Cancer Patients," *Journal of the National Cancer Institute* 85 (1993): 979–987.

24.   See N. Bjurstam, L. Bjorneld, S. W. Duffy, et al., "The Gothenburg Breast Screening Trial: First Results on Mortality, Incidence, and Mode of Detection for Women Ages 39–49 Years at Randomization," *Cancer* 80 (1997): 2091–2099; and J. S. Mandel, J. H. Bond, T. R. Church, et al., "Reducing Mortality from Colorectal Cancer by Screening for Fecal Occult Blood: Minnesota Colon Cancer Control Study," *New England Journal of Medicine* 328 (1993): 1365–1371.

25.   Concerns have been raised that the determination of cause of death was biased in two of the mammography studies: the HIP and one of the Swedish studies. In both cases, it appears that when there was ambiguity, women in the control group were more likely to be labeled a "breast cancer death" than women in the screening group. See O. Olsen and P. C. Gotzsche, "Cochrane Review on Screening for Breast Cancer with Mammography," *Lancet* 358 (2001): 1340–1342; and http://image.thelancet.com/lancet/extra/fullreport.pdf.

26.   This calculation also depends on the baseline rate of death. The more common death is, the easier it is to see a 1 percent change in it. If 10 percent of people are expected to die during the study, for example, over three million people are needed to see a difference; if 20 percent are expected to die, the number drops to around 1.6 million.

27.   Fiscal Year 1999 President's Budget Request. Statement by Dr. Francis S. Collins, Director, National Human Genome Research Institute before the House Subcommittee on Labor, Health and Human Services, Education, and Related Agencies, March 12, 1998.

28.   Although "cancer gene" has become common usage, people don't really have genes for cancer. Instead people have genetic variants that increase the risk of cancer.

29.   I use a single number here for simplicity. It would be more accurate to use a range: somewhere between 40 percent for women with the mutation in the gen-

eral population and 85 percent for women who have the mutation *and* who have already had cancer in the other breast *and* who are from exceptionally high risk families (with at least four members with ovarian or breast cancer diagnosed before the age of 60). See D. Ford, D. F. Easton, D. T. Bishop, et al., and the Breast Cancer Linkage Consortium, "Risks of Cancer in BRCA1-Mutation Carriers," *Lancet* 343 (1994): 692–695; and J. P. Struewing, P. Hartge, S. Wacholder, et al., "The Risk of Cancer Associated with Specific Mutations of BRCA1 and BRCA2 among Ashkenazi Jews," *New England Journal of Medicine* 336 (1997): 1401–1408.

30.   Furthermore, there is reason to wonder just how accurate the risk estimates will be. Early on, most of the risk estimates will come from high-risk families, probably overestimating the true effect of the abnormalities. Later on people who test positive are likely to undergo more subsequent testing than others, which will identify more cancers and thus make the genes, in a sense, a self-fulfilling prophecy. See W. Burke and M. A. Austin, "Genetic Risk in Context: Calculating the Penetrance of BRCA1 and BRCA2 Mutations," *Journal of the National Cancer Institute* 94 (2002): 1185–1187; and C. B. Begg, "On the Use of Familial Aggregation in Population-Based Case Probands for Calculating Penetrance," *Journal of the National Cancer Institute* 94 (2002): 1221–1226.

31.   See L. J. van 't Veer, H. Dai, M. J. van de Vijver, et al., "Gene Expression Profiling Predicts Clinical Outcome of Breast Cancer," *Nature* 415 (2002): 530–536.

CHAPTER 10

1.   Of course, you can get answers to this question in other ways: right now I'm just trying to facilitate a frank discussion with your doctor. But if you want to look further, a good place to start is the U.S. Preventive Services Task Force web site, http://www.ahcpr.gov/clinic/uspstf/uspstopics.htm.

2.   The story of Tommy Thompson's recovery of the SS *Central America*, which sank off the Carolina coast in 1857, is an excellent read. See G. Kinder, *Ship of Gold in the Deep Blue Sea* (New York: Vintage Books, 1999). The importance Thompson attached to independent observations is discussed on page 383.

3.   Useful search terms include *anatomic pathology, surgical pathology, consultations,* and *second opinions.* You might also want to take a look at www.findcancerexperts.com.

4.   S. G. Pauker and J. P. Kassirer, "Contentious Screening Decisions: Does the Choice Matter?" *New England Journal of Medicine* 336 (1997): 1243–1244.

5.   You may be slightly better off having some tests and slightly better off not having others, but for most we really can't make this distinction reliably. With time and more data, this may change.

INDEX

abnormal cells: appearance/organization of, 8, 93–94; body's response to, 174–75, 175 *fig. 17*; confirmatory tests of, 38, 38 *table 2*; DCIS diagnosis of, 101–2, 102 *fig. 14*, 103, 210nn10,12,13; gray zone of, 94–96, 95 *fig. 10*, 103–4; growth rates from, 20–21, 55 *fig. 3*, 200n1; increased detection of, 11, 69–71; lung biopsy of, 91–92; melanoma diagnosis of, 99–101, 99 *fig. 12*, 100 *fig. 13*; nonprogressive types of, 54–56; in Pap smears, 34–35, 41, 49, 202n12; prostate cancer diagnosis of, 96 *fig. 11*, 96–98; second opinion on, 186, 218n3; watchful waiting strategy for, 184, 185–86. *See also* pseudodisease

absolute risk of death: defined, 24, 200n6; personal approaches to, 179–81; with/ without screening, 22–23, 24–26, 200n7. *See also* mortality rate

age adjustment: to incidence rate, 151, 151 *fig. 16*; to mortality rate, 133, 149–50; rationale for, 149

American Cancer Society, 161

ASCUS (atypical squamous cells of unknown significance), 34–35, 41, 202n12

autopsies, 10–11; tissue examination process of, 79–80, 208n19; undiagnosed breast cancer in, 86–88, 87 *table 4*, 208–9n23, 209n24; undiagnosed lung cancer in, 78–79; undiagnosed prostate cancer in, 64, 206nn20,21; undiagnosed thyroid

cancer in, 80–82, 208n20. *See also* pathologists

biopsies: complications from, 45, 203n18; of lung tissue, 91–92; of prostate, 45–46, 74–75; purpose/results of, 35–36; of skin, 142–43, 214n18

bladder cancer, 146–47, 214n22

Blair, Tony, 138

Boston VA Hospital prostate cancer study, 97–98, 103, 209nn4,6,7, 210n13

brain cancer: incidence of, 142; mortality rate for, 147

BRCA1 (breast cancer gene), 170

breast cancer: annual statistics on, 191; diagnostic disagreement on, 101–2, 103, 120 *fig. 14*, 210nn10,12,13; genetic risk for, 170–71, 217nn28,29; genetic testing's assessment of, 173–74; hormonal effects on, 163, 216n19; incidence of, since 1950, 142, 214n16; incidence of early- vs. late-stage, 84–85, 85 *fig. 8*, 86 *fig. 9*, 208n22; increased detection of, 82, 83 *fig. 6*, 208n21, 216n17; missed in screening test, 19–22; mortality rate for, 147, 154–55, 156; number of women tested for, 5, 199n2; pseudodisease form of, 58–59, 204n9; risk factors for, 214n16; screening centers for, 124–25; treatment options for, 82, 83 *fig. 7*; as undiagnosed, in autopsies, 86–88, 87 *table 4*, 208–9n23, 209n24; in

Indexer: Patricia Deminna
Illustrator: Bill Nelson
Compositor: Integrated Composition Systems
Text: 10/14 Palatino
Display: Univers Extended, Bauer Bodoni
Printer and binder: Sheridan Books, Inc.